International College of Person Centered Medicine
Educational Program on Person Centered Care

Seeking the Person
at the Center of Medicine

W. James Appleyard and Juan E. Mezzich
Editors

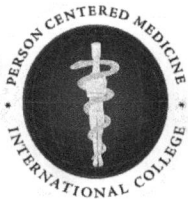

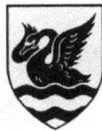

UNIVERSITY OF
BUCKINGHAM
PRESS

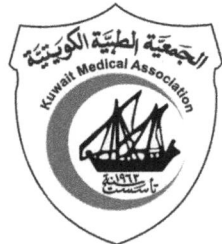

International College of Person Centered Medicine

Educational Program on Person Centered Care

Print ISBN: 9781915054623

E-book ISBN: 9781915054630

Set in Times, Printed by Lightning Source UK

First Edition: 2021

© The University of Buckingham Press Limited 2021

Published by The University of Buckingham Press

51 Gower Street, London WC1E 6HJ

CONTENTS

FOREWORD

As an introduction to this monograph presenting the Educational Program on Person Centered Care from the International College of Person Centered Medicine we would like to list the following objectives of the Program. They have evolved through annual Geneva Conferences and International Congresses [1, 2].

1. To recognise the centrality of the individual person in medical practice and the need for a person and people centred approach to health care.
2. To understand the principles underlying person centred medicine and address strategies and procedures for person-centered care in terms of knowledge, skills and attitudes.
3. To develop skills and attitudes for the person-centered management of clinical problems and health promotion.
4. To understand how the principles underlying person centred care can be renewed in everyday clinical practice for the promotion of wellbeing and within an integrated multi- professional management of Illness.
5. To develop a flexible plan for the implementation, monitoring, evaluation and revision of the educational program.

The person has always been in the center of medicine and medical developments but in the language in current use of patients involved in healthcare *Individuals* are labelled in different ways which are descriptive not of a person but of a relationship and likely never will reflect the wide diversity of each individual. That is why the prefix person centered has become so important.

Historically early communities were simple and skills and knowledge were basic. With a sick person those around waited and watched for a resolution of illness and probably comforted others when they could others. With few therapeutic measures available, magical healing as accompaniment by the 'medicine man' and the family became key features.

The mutation into a physician depended on observation , the accumulation of knowledge, records and eventually the development of a structure within society with apprenticeship, centres of learning and places where treatment could be delivered by specialists. Trade Guilds emerged which controlled the way in which physicians were able to practice.

The torch of medical learning was not passed on smoothly like a relay baton but with the emergence of Islam in 7th Century CE, Greek and Roman texts were translated into Arabic, incorporating the wisdom and practices from many centuries and from many civilizations stretching Westward from China. Physicians such as Haroon Al Rashid, Rhazes and Avicenna residing in Bagdad were prominent in the Eastern Arab Caliphate between 766 and 1,037CE.

The Islamic invasion of the Iberian Peninsula in 711CE took this wealth of knowledge to Northern Europe. Physicians who emerged here and flourished included Avenzoar and Maimonides. European medicine was therefore led out of the Dark Ages as a result of communication with the Arab world. Europe continued to benefit enormously from the wealth of medical knowledge brought by Islam via Spain.   Therapies not practised in Europe and a knowledge of herbal medicine was part of this legacy. In addition, the Arab influence left behind important principles of care such as that of incorporating centres of treatment into communities with Barristan's courtyards with medical facilities as well as places of commerce and refuge. Many of their traditional principles in the delivery of care such as holistic treatment, specialist units, outreach home visits, annual accreditation, multi-professional care and a minimum of religious control are being refreshed by the person centered movement.

Evolving in parallel with person-centered care, evidence-based medicine arrived as a 'new approach to teaching the practice of medicine, advanced as the 'new paradigm' for medical practice. It de-emphasized intuition, unsystematic clinical experience and pathophysiology as adequate grounds for clinical decision-making, recommending instead the use of purely 'scientific' evidence. However, it is the person as a patient who must exercise the final choice. Thus, a healthcare system which mandates the use of rigid 'evidence-based' guidelines has the potential to lead directly to a 'misaligning of the goals of doctors and patients'.

It has become clear that reductionist models of health care are unsustainable in both economic and humanistic terms. There is a pressing need, therefore, articulated increasingly by patients themselves, to move away from impersonal, fragmented and decontextualized systems of healthcare towards personalized, integrated and contextualised models of clinical practice within a humanistic framework of care that recognizes the importance of applying science in a manner which respects the patient as a whole person and takes full account of his values, preferences, aspirations stories, cultural context, fears, worries and hopes and which thus recognizes and responds to his emotional, social and spiritual necessities in addition to his physical needs.

The Educational Program for Person-centered Care aims to achieve this. It is divided into three discrete but interrelated sections. The first section of four papers includes the conceptualization and measurement in person centered medicine and embraces the relevance of the social determinants of health and people centered public health. The second group of articles moves on to the practical aspects of patient-physician communication and the importance of a comprehensive diagnosis. The third section emphasizes the importance of shared decision making with key examples and inter-professional collaboration. The program is a living document and will be revised with the help of those who study and apply a person-centered approach to their own practice.

W. James Appleyard and Juan E. Mezzich, Editors.

REFERENCES

1. ICPCM. Zagreb Declaration 2013 on Person-centered Professional Education. Int J Person Centered Medicine 4: 6-7, 2014.
2. ICPCM. Madrid Declaration 2016 on Medical Education and the Goals of Health Care. Int J Person Centered Medicine 7: 80-81, 2017.

PREFACE

This excellent treatise covers extensive work by internationally recognized active and practicing clinicians who are members of the International College of Person-Centered Medicine. It is a crucial and indispensable subject for every health practitioner and persons involved in health care systems.

The first section focuses on Medical Professionalism, Ethical and Human Rights Foundations of Person-Centered Medicine, a person-Centered Approach by Physicians and the Concepts and Strategies of People-Centered Public Health.

The second section addresses the importance of Clinical Communication and empathy for Collaborative Care and discusses the concepts and procedures for Person-centered integrative diagnosis for a Person-Centered Assessment and Care across the lifecycle.

The last section highlights the importance of care planning and inter-disciplinary team decision making especially in mental and comorbid conditions, oncology cases, palliative Care, and other general conditions adequately in a person and people-centered way. This section also addresses the need for Inter-Professional Collaboration as a means for a broader person-centered perspective in medicine.

This book presents an authoritative overview of the person-centered educational journey. Written by experts in the respective fields, the text covers the concepts and strategies focusing on ethical commitment, a holistic approach, relationship focus, cultural awareness and responsiveness, individualized care, establishment of mutual trust and understanding between the patients, their families and clinicians for shared clinical decision making and offering people-centered healthcare service delivery.

As an invaluable companion and resource for all involved in clinical care, the book will be especially welcomed by primary care physicians, social workers, and every medical professional.

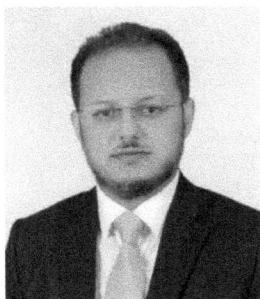

Dr. Ahmed Thuwaini Al-Enizi
President of KMA

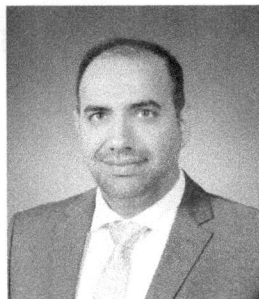

Dr. Salem Ali Al-Kandari
Secretary General of KMA

SECTION 1

General Concepts and Organization

EDITORIAL INTRODUCTION

ICPCM EDUCATIONAL PROGRAM ON PERSON CENTERED CARE: GENERAL CONCEPTS AND ORGANIZATION

W. James Appleyard, MA, MD, FRCP[a] and
Juan E. Mezzich, MD, MA, MSc, PhD[b]

Keywords: person-centered medicine, educational program, person-centered care, International College of Person Centered Medicine

Correspondence Address: Prof. W. James Appleyard, Thimble Hall Blean Common, Kent CT2 9JJ, United Kingdom

E-mail: jimappleyard2510@aol.com

INTRODUCTION TO THE ICPCM EDUCATIONAL PROGRAM ON PERSON CENTERED CARE

The International College of Person Centered Medicine's Educational program is being developed in collaboration with our colleagues from the Indian Medical Association from a series of three symposia held during the ICPCM's 6th International Congress of Person Centered Medicine in New Delhi, 2018. The purpose of the program is to spread understanding of the principles underlying person-centered medicine and to address strategies and procedures for person-centered care in terms of knowledge, skills, and attitudes [1].

---

[a] Board Advisor and Former President, International College of Person Centered Medicine; Former President, World Medical Association; Former President, International Association of Medical Colleges

[b] Professor of Psychiatry, Icahn School of Medicine at Mount Sinai, New York, USA; Hipólito Unanue Chair of Person Centered Medicine, San Marcos National University, Lima; Former President, World Psychiatric Association; Former President and Current Secretary General, International College of Person Centered Medicine; Editor, International Journal of Person Centered Medicine

The program emphasizes the centrality of the individual person in medical practice and the need for a person- and people-centered approach to health care [2]. To achieve this goal, medical professionalism within an interprofessional environment, which is based on values inherent in medical ethics and human rights forms the foundations of person-centered care [3]. The skills and attitudes developed for the person-centered management of clinical problems and health promotion need to be renewed in everyday clinical practice for the promotion of well-being and the management of illness [4].

Health systems have fragmented and depersonalized clinical care, subjecting it to heavy commercialization and bureaucratization, depending on the country. Increased specialization has given rise to narrower medical subspecialties. There is a growing dissatisfaction among the medical profession with their professional role [5]. As a consequence of this "hyper-technification" there is a major "scientistic" reduction in medical care, which tends to distance doctors from giving care rooted in genuinely human encounters and many doctors experience a loss of meaning in their work life. Such professional burnout, affecting the emotions, mentality, behavior, and sociability of doctors, has a proven negative impact on work teams and patient care. At the same time, the public health is being endangered by new infectious, environmental, and behavioral threats superimposed upon rapid demographic and epidemiological transitions. As health systems struggle to keep up with demand and are becoming more complex and costlier, additional stress is placed on health workers.

In many countries, professionals are encountering more socially diverse patients with chronic conditions, who are more proactive in their health-seeking behavior. Patient management requires coordinated care across time and space, demanding unprecedented teamwork. Professionals have to integrate the explosive growth of knowledge and technologies while grappling with expanding functions – super-specialization, prevention, and complex care management in many sites, including different types of facilities alongside home-based and community-based care [6]. In addition to the rapid pace of change in health, there is a parallel revolution in education. The explosive increase not only in total volume of information, but also in ease of access to it, means that the role of universities and other educational institutions needs to be rethought [7]. Learning, of course, has always been experienced outside formal instruction through all types of interactions, but the informational content and learning potential are today without precedent. In this rapidly evolving context, universities and educational institutions are broadening their traditional role as places where people go to obtain information (e.g., by consulting books in libraries or listening to expert faculty members) and to incorporate novel forms of learning that transcend the confines of the classroom. The new generations of learners need the capacity to discriminate vast amounts of information and extract and synthesize knowledge that is necessary for clinical and population-based decision making. These developments point toward new opportunities for the methods, means, and meaning of a person-centered medical education [8].

The language we use of patient involvement in health care is important. Currently it is both confusing and controversial. Language transmits values and beliefs, reflecting and shaping social perceptions and power relationships. In the current use of the language of patient involvement in health care, individuals are labeled in different ways, which are descriptive not *of a person* but *of a relationship* and likely never will reflect the wide diversity of each individual. That is why the prefix *person centered* is so important.

The word *patient* is limited in its descriptiveness. By definition a patient is "a sufferer – one who suffers patiently and one who is under medical treatment". This implies a lack of autonomy, passivity, and dependency [9]. The words people use to describe themselves reflect their relationship with their illness or disability and can therefore have personal and emotional significance.

In the United Kingdom, the terms "user," "service user," consumer, and client have increasingly replaced "patient" in relation to involvement in health and social care service delivery, research, or education. Service user, however, defines a person by a single narrow aspect of their life (using a specific service) and can be pejorative, demeaning, and stigmatizing. It neglects those who do not or cannot access services, and it does not devolve power or respect to the people who use services. Many "patients" or "service users" involved in health professional education are not ill or currently receiving medical care. The prefix "lay" defines people in terms of who or what they are *not* (e.g., a professional). It implies a lack of expertise when many patients will themselves be experts in their own illnesses.

Person-centered medicine does not recognize an obligation to care for their "patient's" solely on their own terms – the clinician just being a provider of goods – but rather within the context of two people, the person as a patient and the physician as a person engage in a dialogical process of shared decision making focused on the patient as a person, and his or her best interests, in a caring atmosphere within a relationship of engagement, trust, and responsibility.

The two foundational components of medical practice, the science and the art of medicine, should be applied within an ethical and humanistic framework [10]. There is therefore a need to move toward more personalized, integrated, and contextualized models of clinical practice with the active involvement of "patients" as persons, and with members of their families.

Current *evidence-based medicine* overemphasizes the value of scientific standardization, its compartmentalism of knowledge, fragmentation of services, and relative neglect of patients' personal concerns, needs, and values, while *patient-centered medicine* overemphasizes patient's choice. In contrast, *person-centered medicine*, with its biological, social, psychological, and spiritual model brings both science and art together. Person-centered medicine ensures that patients are known as persons in the context of their own social worlds, listened to, informed, respected, and involved in their care and having their wishes honored during their health care journey.

Person-centered care fosters a feeling of connectedness with an interpersonal outlook of unity, which promotes attitudes of hope, empathy, and respect. One of the key aspects of clinical care is reaching a diagnosis in its widest sense, which provides the fundamental basis for planning therapy and care. The *person-centered integrative diagnosis model* is designed to do this [11]. It assesses informational domains of both ill and positive aspects of health on a three-level schema – the first is the health status, the second the experience of health and illness, and the third the contributors to health and illness. With an enhancement of well-being, the rates of relapse and recurrence of physical and mental disorders tend to be reduced.

PROGRAM ORGANIZATION

The structure of the ICPCM educational program on person-centered care involves three components. The first one corresponds to general concepts of person-centered medicine and the organization of the educational program. The second component involves communication, interviewing, and comprehensive diagnosis. And the third component involves care planning and shared decision making in general and in major conditions as well as interprofessional collaboration and health services organization.

INTRODUCING THE PAPERS IN THIS SECTION OF THE MONOGRAPH

The present section of the monograph is dedicated to the first set of the educational program.

In the first article, Person Centered Medicine Foundations for Medical Education, Mezzich et al. trace the ICPCM's institutional journey that, from its beginning, was defined as an approach that places the person in context as the center of health and as the goal of health care. As a theory of medicine, and in contrast to reductionist perspectives, person-centeredness involves medicine informed by evidence, experience, and values, and oriented to promote the health and well-being of the whole person [12]. Through a critical review of the literature and broad international consultation, a study on the systematic conceptualization and measurement of PCM was undertaken by the International College of Person Centered Medicine with support from the World Health Organization [13].

This elucidated the key concepts of PCM to be (1) Ethical Commitment, (2) Cultural Awareness and Responsiveness, (3) Holistic Approach, (4) Relational Focus, (5) Individualization of Care, (6) Common Ground for Collaborative Diagnosis and Shared Decision Making, (7) People-Centered Organization of Services, and (8) Person-Centered Education and Research.

The collegial environment of the ICPCM fosters collaboration at all levels, creativity and the development of ideas through its annual Geneva Conferences and also annual International Congresses in different world locations [14].

In the second article on "Medical Professionalism and Ethical and Human Rights Foundations of Person Centered Medicine," Snaedal argues that humanistic and scientific medicine must take into consideration the whole person, whether healthy or during disease, as well as his or her family and immediate surroundings. It is thus inherently centered on the person [15] and it must be based on general ethical and human rights as declared in various international documents. As the foundations of medical professionalism and competence, it is of profound importance for successful outcomes in health care [16]. The policies adopted by the World Medical Association (WMA) representing more than 9 million physicians worldwide are therefore having a central role in physicians' everyday work and their ethical conduct [17].

One of the first policies to be adopted by the WMA when it was founded in 1948 after World War II, was the physician's oath or pledge named the Declaration of Geneva (DoG) [18]. The pledge is still considered to be the modern version of the Hippocratic Oath and is intended to be addressed to and accepted by medical students when they enter the profession. The WMA Declaration of Seoul on Professional Autonomy states that professional autonomy and clinical independence are core elements of medical professionalism and are essential for the delivery of high-quality health care and therefore benefit patients and society. The WMA laid out the basis for the rights of patients in its Declaration of Lisbon [19]. In its preamble it is stated: "while a physician should always act according to his/her conscience, and always in the best interests of the patient, equal effort must be made to guarantee patient autonomy and justice."

As Person-centered medicine is inherently centered on the person in contrast to evidence-based medicine (EBM) that to great extent focuses on standardized groups, it is broadly consistent with policies adopted by the United Nations (UN) and the World Medical Association (WMA).

The third paper on "The Making of a Physician: A Person-Centered Approach" by Sharma and Sharma from New Delhi emphasizes that the essence of medicine lies in the therapeutic relationship between the doctor and the patient as a person in totality in both health and disease. The relief of suffering and the cure of a person must be seen as the twin obligations of the profession with true dedication to the cure of the sick. The cure of disease is influenced by our scientific knowledge and growth of an evidence base, while the relief of suffering is guided by our compassion and consolation skills.

There is no such thing as valueless medicine. All physicians in medicine practice need to carry shared professional values, standards, aims, and goals over their lifetime of medical practice. The value of human life is to be respected whether patients are in the developed or developing countries. In Sharma and Sharma's view the final answer lies in the conscience of the doctor, a universal respect for human values, and the ideology of humanism. There is an urgent need to incorporate and reemphasize "value" and "compassion" in the care of patients within medical education and integrating person-centered care into daily medical practice. An ethical and value-based approach must also be regarded as an essential part of health service management.

In the fourth paper on "Concepts and Strategies of People-Centered Public Health" Canchihuaman et al. contend that in order to improve public health worldwide a people-centered approach is needed. Since public health and clinical medicine might be seen as two sides of the same coin, their values and principles are equivalent applicable [20] but some special considerations for public health requires to be taken due to its particular nature.

The person-centered approach establishes its bases in an equilibrium that must exist between the liberty (individual's right to liberty) and solidarity (the obligation for protecting individual's welfare). Other principles and values mentioned were: equity, social justice, sustainable development and holistic conception of persons. Public health inspired by people-centered public health approach may result in a wider scope of action and more efficient functions' performance; for example by undertaking integral strategies for "enhancing prevention, promotion, protection, and prolonging life", placing at the front of goals to address social and environmental determinants of health or developing sustained, continuous, and integrated services for the different stages of people's lives. Ultimately, it promotes sustainable development through the articulation of public health and primary care within universal health coverage [21].

ACKNOWLEDGMENTS AND DISCLOSURES

The authors have no conflicts of interest to report concerning this paper.

REFERENCES

1. Mezzich JE, Appleyard J, Botbol M. 2017. Engagement and Empowerment in Person Centered Medicine. International Journal of Person Centered Medicine 7 (1): 1–4.
2. Mezzich JE, Snaedal J, van Weel C, Botbol M, Salloum I. 2011. Introduction to Person-Centered Medicine: From Concepts to Practice. Journal of Evaluation in Clinical Practice 17 (2): 330–332.
3. Desai K, Appleyard J. 2017. Human Rights and Person Centered Medicine: The Need of the Hour. International Journal of Person Centered Medicine 7 (3): 161–164.
4. Deau X, Appleyard J. 2015. Person Centered Medicine as an Ethical Imperative. International Journal of Person-Centered Medicine 5 (2): 60–63.
5. Appleyard J, Botbol M, Caballero F, Ghebrehiwet T, Mezzich JE, Perez-Miranda J, Ruiz-Moral R, Salloum IM, Snaedal J, Van Leberghe W. 2017. Bases of Person Centered Medical Education to Enhance Health Systems Worldwide. International Journal of Person Centered Medicine 7 (2): 82–90.
6. Ghebrehiwet T. 2013. Effectiveness of Team Approach in Health Care: Some Research Evidence. International Journal of Person Centered Medicine 3 (2): 137–139.
7. Madrid Declaration on Medical Education and the Goals of Health Care. International Journal of Person Centered Medicine 2016.
8. Zagreb Declaration on Person-Centered Professional Education. International Journal of Person Centered Medicine 2013.
9. Appleyard J. 2014. An Introduction to Person Centered Medicine. ICPCM Newsletter. personcenteredmedicine.org
10. Miles A, Mezzich JE. 2011. The Care of the Patient and the Soul of the Clinic: Person-Centered Medicine as an Emergent Model of Modern Clinical Practice. International Journal of Person Centered Medicine 1 (2): 207–222.
11. Wallcraft J, Amering M, Steffen S, Salloum IM. 2012. Evaluators and Assessment Process in Person-Centred Integrative Diagnosis. International Journal of Person Centered Medicine 2 (2): 201–204.
12. Mezzich JE, Snaedal J, van Weel C, Heath I (eds). 2010. Conceptual Explorations on Person-Centered Medicine. International Journal of Integrated Care (Suppl 10).
13. Mezzich JE, Kirisci L, Salloum IM, Trivedi JK, Kar SK, Adams N, Wallcraft J. 2016. Systematic Conceptualization of Person Centered Medicine and Development and Validation of a Person-Centered Care Index. International Journal of Person Centered Medicine 6: 219–247.

14. Mezzich J. 2012. The Construction of Person-Centered Medicine and the Launching of an International College. International Journal of Person Centered Medicine 2 (1): 6–10.
15. Mezzich J, Snaedal J, van Weel C, Heath I. 2010. Toward Person-Centered Medicine: From Disease to Patient to Person. Mount Sinai Journal of Medicine 77 (3): 304–306.
16. Epstein RM, Hundert EM. 2002. Defining and Assessing Professional Competence. Journal of the American Medical Association 287 (2): 226–235.
17. https://www.wma.net/policies-post/wma-international-code-of-medical-ethics
18. https://www.wma.net/policies-post/wma-declaration-of-geneva
19. https://www.wma.net/policies-post/wmadeclaration-of-lisbon-on-the-rights-of-the-patient
20. Appleyard J, Botbol M, Epperly T, Ghebrehiwet T, Grove J, Mezzich JE, Rawaf S, Salloum IM, Snaedal J, Van Dulmen S. 2016. Patterns and Prospects for the Implementation of Person-Centered Primary Care and People-Centered Public Health. International Journal of Person Centered Medicine 6 (1): 9–17.
21. White F. 2015. Primary Health Care and Public Health: Foundations of Universal Health Systems. Medical Principles and Practice 24 (2): 103–116.

PERSON CENTERED MEDICINE FOUNDATIONS FOR MEDICAL EDUCATION

Juan E. Mezzich, MD, MA, MSc, PhD[a], Ihsan Salloum, MD, MPH[b], Levent Kirisci, PhD[c], and Alberto Perales, MD, DMSc, Dipl-Ethics, MSc[d]

ABSTRACT

Background: The development of person-centered medical education is inscribed within an international programmatic movement toward a medicine focused on the totality of the person. This movement, with broad historical bases, has been maturing since 2008 through conferences with global health institutions, research projects, and academic publications. A key challenge in the application of person-centered medicine (PCM) to the practice of medicine has been the elucidation of its core principles and the development of operationalized measures that allows for assessment of the degree of person-centeredness in clinical care and medical education.
Objectives: The aim of this paper is to elucidate the core principles of what is currently understood as PCM in order to inform the development of medical education programs.
Methods: In order to elucidate the core PCM concepts, the following main approaches were employed: A systematic review of the literature and consultation exercises with broad international panels of health professionals and representatives of patient and family organizations. A Person-Centered Care Index (PCI) was then developed from identified core concepts and its acceptability, reliability, and validity were tested in three international sites, California, USA; London, England;

[a] Professor of Psychiatry, Icahn School of Medicine at Mount Sinai, New York, USA; Hipolito Unanue Professor of Person Centered Medicine, San Fernando Faculty of Medicine, San Marcos National University, Lima, Peru; Secretary General, International College of Person Centered Medicine; Former President, World Psychiatric Association
[b] Professor of Psychiatry, University of Miami Medical School, Miami, FL, USA; Board Director, International College of Person Centered Medicine
[c] Professor of Pharmaceutical Sciences, University of Pittsburgh, Pittsburgh, Pennsylvania, USA; Statistical Editor, International Journal of Person Centered Medicine
[d] Extraordinary Expert Professor and Professor of Psychiatry, San Fernando Faculty of Medicine, San Marcos National University, Lima, Peru; Former President, National Academy of Medicine, Lima, Peru; Former President, Latin American Network of Person-Centered Medicine

and Lucknow, India. Reflection exercises were then conducted among the authors to outline strategies and activities to organize medical education programs.

Results: The following eight key principles of PCM were identified: (1) Ethical Commitment; (2) Cultural Awareness and Responsiveness; (3) Holistic Approach; (4) Relational Focus; (5) Individualization of Care; (6) Common Ground for Collaborative Diagnosis and Shared Decision Making; (7) People-Centered Organization of Services; and (8) Person-Centered Education and Research. The PCI validation showed high internal consistency, unidimensionality through factor analysis, and substantial interrater reliability, acceptability, and content validity.

Discussion: The presented principles and strategies are consistent with suggestions offered in the literature and may serve as bases for the design of educational programs and research instruments. Their continuous refinement is proposed through future international and local studies to clarify the key concepts of the movement as well as strategies for their practical clinical application.

Conclusions: The elucidation of key concepts of person-centered health care has provided further clarity to the field on the key ingredients for the practice of person-centered medicine. The PCI provides an operationalized measure to assess the degree of person-centeredness in health care services and medical education and heralds a new paradigm for measuring optimized, person-centered care models.

Keywords: clinical care, person, concepts, principles, strategies, clinical activities, medical education, person-centered medicine

Correspondence: Prof. Juan E. Mezzich, Icahn School of Medicine at Mount Sinai, Fifth Ave & 100 St., Box 1093, New York, New York 10029, USA

E-mail: juanmezzich@aol.com

INTRODUCTION

The development of a person-centered clinical care is part of the international programmatic movement aimed at placing the whole person and its context in the center of health and as a goal of health services. Consequently, this article will first briefly review the bases of a person-centered medicine and, later, the process of development of the corresponding international programmatic movement.

The objectives, methods, and results of a project of elucidation of the key concepts that underlie person-centered medicine and the subsequent strategy approach for the implementation of the enunciated principles will be delineated.

18

These achievements and approaches will be discussed in the context of similar efforts, their value for the construction of evaluative instruments will be examined, and future studies will be outlined to reinforce and refine the presented approaches.

Bases of a Person-Centered Medicine and Health

The development of modern medicine has facilitated important scientific advances in the understanding of diseases and their implications for diagnosis and treatment, as well as the prolongation of life expectancy. Such modern development, at the same time, has favored a conceptual reductionism, hyperbolic attention to the organ and the disease, professional super-specialization, fragmentation of the clinical attention, conversion of the acts of service into salable products [1, 2], trivializing the doctor–patient relationship and distancing it from solidarity and respect for human dignity, and interfering with a vocation of service to people who need help.

In response to these limitations and deviations, an international movement has emerged that seeks to reprioritize the totality of the person as the center of medicine and health in line with the earliest roots of medicine found in the ancient Asian and Hellenic civilizations, which tended to conceptualize health broadly and holistically [3–5]. In this same line, the concept of health in pre-Columbian medicine establishes a fundamental balance between the physical, social, and spiritual dimensions of the person, in which moderation in diet, exercise, and appropriate behavior are considered essential for a healthy life [6, 7]. These historical notions are reflected in the comprehensive definition of health inscribed in the constitution of the World Health Organization as "a state of complete physical, mental and social well-being and not merely the absence of disease" [8].

In Peru, Honorio Delgado [9] pointed out in his "Physician, Medicine and Soul," the following: "Positivism, abusive generalization of ideas valid only in the domain of the physical sciences, leads to consider the patient as a material object, a thing, and medicine as a pure science or a mixture of science and technique, therefore, impersonal and mechanical." Carlos Alberto Seguín [10, 11] proposed a radical change where doctors would not be "veterinarians of human beings" but "men dealing with men." Seguín emphasized in his medical teachings the essential importance of the human bond with the patient.

Programmatic Development of Person-Centered Medicine

The conceptualization and development of a medicine and health centered on the person and the community [12–15] have been maturing through the Geneva Conferences on Person Centered Medicine carried out annually since 2008 in collaboration with the World Health Organization, the World Medical Association, the International Council of Nurses and the International Alliance of Patient Organizations, and the company of around 30 global health institutions, and from which an International College of Person Centered Medicine has emerged. The academic support of this international movement can be illustrated with the International Journal of Person Centered Medicine, published in collaboration with Buckingham University Press [16] and a forthcoming textbook on Person Centered Psychiatry published by Springer [17] as well as like, under the auspices of important universities of Europe and the Americas to the mentioned events, and with the recently established Latin American Network of Person-Centered Medicine [18] that in joint effort with the National Academy of Medicine of Peru and other Academies of Medicine of the Region has been holding Latin American Conferences in this field.

This new global initiative articulates science and humanism toward a medicine *of* the person (and their total health, from disease to quality of life), *for* the person (promoting the fulfillment of each person's life project), *from* the person (cultivating the health professional as a person, with high ethical and scientific aspirations), and *with* the person (respectfully collaborating with the person who appears in search of help) [13, 19]. It is therefore a medicine where science is an essential instrument and humanism its very essence.

OBJECTIVES

The information on historical precedents and clinical and public health challenges summarized above provides indications and perspectives relevant to the conceptualization of person-centered medicine. Such understanding can be optimized through efforts toward a systematization of prevalent and pertinent notions. The International College of Person Centered Medicine (ICPCM) has taken up this endeavor through presentations and discussions at the Geneva Conferences since 2008 [20, 21]. More recently, this institutional concern of the ICPCM has been embodied in a project on the systematic conceptualization of person-centered care and the measurement of advances in this field, with the support of the World Health Organization [22]. Based on such project, this article aims to elucidate the conceptual principles of person-centered medicine and then delineate strategies for its practical application in clinical care services.

METHODS

The achievement of the mentioned objectives has been based on literature reviews, international consultations, and reflection on indices and guidelines obtained. These approaches are briefly described below, largely constituted by the methodology of the ICPCM project mentioned above. The detailed presentation of the ICPCM study and its different aspects is made in another publication [23].

Systematic Review of the Literature

The review of the literature around the bases of health care focused on the person and the community was carried out in two phases. The first focused on the presentations made at the Geneva Conferences on Person Centered Medicine from 2008 to 2010, the articles available on these papers in the archives of the International College of Person Centered Medicine, and the additional literature from members of advisory groups. The second phase involved a search of the Pub Med information banks of the United States National Library of Medicine in subsequent years. The results of the review of the 70 pertinent articles found were tabulated to facilitate the identification of patterns and indices. The tabulated information included: authors and date, title of the publication, summary of results, and key ideas [23].

International Consultation

This consultation involved two broad international groups. The central group working closely with the project directors through teleconferences was made up of 17 experts from the Americas, Europe, Africa, Asia, and Oceania, including doctors from multiple specialties, as well as representatives of nurses, social workers, patients, and family members. The second group involved a broad panel consisting of 56 international experts from all continents, including doctors and other health professionals, both clinicians and researchers. This panel was consulted through e-mails.

The first phase of the International Consultation involved the discussion and evaluation of the tabulated review of the literature by the central group. The task assigned to this group was to identify in the tabulated literature a set of descriptive key areas of health services focused on the person and the community. This set included a first group of 14 areas related to "Personal Health Care" and another one of seven areas related to "Public Health and Service Organization." More specifically, the first group of areas looked person centered, while the second group focused on the community. Next, the areas obtained from the literature were organized in a form to facilitate their examination and processing by the broad panel. The final section of the form offered space to list additional conceptual areas drawn from the literature by the panelists themselves. Panelists were also asked to rate the importance (high, medium, or low) of each of the areas listed to describe person-centered care, as well as to delineate within each area crucial elements to characterize person-centered care and community.

The next phase of the International Consultation involved the analysis, by the central group, of the evaluation forms produced by the broad panel in order to design, in collaboration with the study directors, a Person-Centered Care Index (PCI).

Reflection toward Practical Strategies

The directors of the original study conducted reflection sessions to weigh the results of the consultations and the emerging Person-Centered Care Index. A more recent purpose of reflection has been to identify promising strategies for the implementation of the principles of person-centered medicine toward a person-centered clinical care and medical education.

RESULTS

Formulation of Principles of Person-Centered Medicine

Based on the aforementioned review of the literature, international consultations, and weighted reflection, the following eight key concepts or principles of person-centered medicine were identified:

- Ethical Commitment
- Cultural Awareness and Responsiveness
- Holistic Approach
- Relational Focus
- Individualization of Care
- Common Ground for Collaborative Diagnosis and Shared Decision Making
- People-Centered Organization of Services
- Person-Centered Education and Research

Each of these key concepts contains a series of denotations and connotations that help explain their meaning, implications, and scope. They come from the process of reviewing the literature, international consultations, and thoughtful reflection. Its detailed specification has been presented by Mezzich, Kirisci et al [23].

Design of a Person-Centered Care Index

The ICPCM study directors, with the comments of the central group of international consultants mentioned above, set out to design a prototype index that allows the evaluation of progress toward a focus on the person and the community. With this objective, the eight key concepts accepted as major indices were used. It was considered that the first six corresponded to individual clinical care, while the last two referred to general health systems and their support activities. The key concepts or major indices were found related to a set of subconcepts that added 33 subindices. It was postulated that the presence of each of these indices and subindices in a given service or health system could be qualified in terms of its frequency using a 4-point scale (1 = never, 2 = sometimes, 3 = frequently, and 4 = always). In addition, it was proposed that to achieve a global average score, the partial scores are added and the result is divided among the number of items that could have been evaluated. It was also agreed to have a blank space at the end of the format for additional narrative comments.

Figure 1 shows the English version of the Person-Centered Care Index (PCI).

Practical Strategies for Person-Centered Care and Education

The formulation of practical strategies for person-centered care and professional education as implementation of the principles of person-centered medicine also revealed a series of more specific concepts of denotative or connotative nature that were used for the design of the Person-Centered Care Index. From this process and the weighted reflection mentioned above, a series of proposals emerge as practical strategies for person-centered care. These are presented below, in Table 1, displayed next to each of the key concepts or principles of person-centered medicine with the hope they facilitate their practical implementation for health care and professional training.

DISCUSSION

Both the key concepts and the practical strategies presented in this article are consistent with observations and suggestions in recent literature. For example, Leyns & De Maeseneer [25] obtained similar results particularly applied to primary health care. An international survey conducted by Harding [26] on person-centered care showed that this perspective is widely present in the health policies of most English-speaking countries, although with a great delay in its implementation.

There is also a substantive consistency between the concepts and strategies listed in this article with the information fields and procedural aspects of the model of Person-Centered Integrative Diagnosis (PID) [27]. Indeed, its components clearly include most of the principles and strategies mentioned above. The PID model has been applied in the Latin American Guide to Psychiatric Diagnosis, Revised Version (GLADP-VR) [28], whose use in this world region has been growing. Already the first edition of the Latin American Guide (GLADP) [29] had

Person-centered Care Index

Please rate the following person-centered care indicators in terms of their level of presence in a given health system. To obtain a global average PCI score, please add the partial scores and divide this by the number of items actually rated.

N°	Indicators	Not Present	Moderately Present	Substantially Present	Highly Present
1.	**Ethical Framework**				
1.1	Respect for the dignity of every person involved	1	2	3	4
1.2	Respect for the patient's rights	1	2	3	4
1.3	Promoting the patient's autonomy	1	2	3	4
1.4	Promoting the patient's empowerment	1	2	3	4
1.5	Promoting the fulfillment of the patient's life project	1	2	3	4
1.6	Attending to the patient's personal values and needs	1	2	3	4
2	**Cultural Sensitivity**				
2.1	Attending to the patient's ethnic identity and values	1	2	3	4
2.2	Attending to the patient's language needs	1	2	3	4
2.3	Attending to the patient's gender needs	1	2	3	4
2.4	Attending to the patient's spiritual needs	1	2	3	4
3.	**Holistic Approach**				
3.1	Utilizing a bio-psycho-socio-cultural-spiritual framework	1	2	3	4
3.2	Attending to both ill-health (diseases, disabilities) and positive health or well-being (functioning, resilience, resources, and quality of life)	1	2	3	4
4.	**Relational Focus**				
4.1	Cultivating the clinician–patient relationship	1	2	3	4
4.2	Displaying empathy in clinical communication and the care process	1	2	3	4
4.3	Cultivating trust during clinical communication and the care process	1	2	3	4
5.	**Individualization of Care**				
5.1	Attending to the patient's uniqueness	1	2	3	4

Figure 1. Person-Centered Care Index

5.2	Attending to the patient's evolving situation	1	2	3	4
5.3	Attending to the patient's context	1	2	3	4
5.4	Attending to the patient's personal choices	1	2	3	4
6.	**Organization and Implementation of Person-Centered Care**				
6.1	Promoting shared understanding of the patient's health situation	1	2	3	4
6.2	Conducting personalized diagnosis	1	2	3	4
6.3	Shared decision making for treatment planning and the care process	1	2	3	4
7.	**People-Centered Organization of Services**				
7.1	Advocacy for the health and rights of all people in the community	1	2	3	4
7.2	People's participation in the planning of health services	1	2	3	4
7.3	Promoting partnership at all levels of service organization	1	2	3	4
7.4	Promoting quality of personalized services	1	2	3	4
7.5	Service responsiveness to community needs and expectations	1	2	3	4
7.6	Integration and coordination of services around the patient's needs	1	2	3	4
7.7	Emphasis on people-centered primary care	1	2	3	4
7.8	Attentiveness to international perspectives and developments for person-centered care	1	2	3	4
8.	**Person-Centered Education, Training, and Research**				
8.1	Promoting person-centered public health education	1	2	3	4
8.2	Promoting person-centered health professional training	1	2	3	4
8.3	Promoting person-centered clinical research	1	2	3	4
Global average score					
Additional evaluative comments:					

Figure 1. (*Continued*)

been favorably compared with the DSM-IV of the American Psychiatric Association and the International Classification of Diseases of the World Health Organization since it was considered more holistic and culturally sensitive by psychiatrists in the region [30].

Table 1. Principles and Strategies for Person-Centered Clinical Care and Medical Education

Principles of Person-Centered Medicine	Strategies for Person-Centered Clinical Care and Medical Education
Ethical Commitment	• Respect for the dignity of the person • Recognition of the autonomy and responsibility of the person in the care of their health. • Informed consent as a dialogical ethical process • Promotion of the life project of every person involved
Cultural Awareness and Responsiveness	• Awareness on cultural diversity (ancestry and current context) with which the patient identifies, as well a student and teacher • Attention and respect for the patient's cultural explanations about his or her health and illness • Clinicians' awareness of their own cultural identity • Integrative response in the diagnosis and therapeutic plans to the cultural identities of the patient and the clinicians
Holistic Approach	• Attention to the biological, psychological, social, economic, ecological, cultural, and spiritual aspects of the disease • Attention to such aspects regarding positive health and well-being • Specific attention to the family context in the understanding of the health status of the person and in restorative and promotional health actions • Consideration of the total and interactively dynamic integrity of the person in context
Relational Focus	• Establish empathy as a key communication support for care and education • Facilitate that the patient expresses everything he or she wants to express • Listen to the patient attentively, with "more than two ears" [24] attuned to their conscious and subconscious subjectivity and narrative • Consideration of the ethical relationship of service between the clinician and the patient • Cultivate communication and effective relationships with the family and the team of professionals involved
Individualization of Care	• Consideration of the individual's biological, psychological, and social particular profile • Consideration of their risk factors and protective factors of health • Consideration of experience, values, and preferences • Delineation of an individualized program for care

Table 1. (*Continued*)

Principles of Person-Centered Medicine	Strategies for Person-Centered Clinical Care and Medical Education
Common Ground for Collaborative Diagnosis and Shared Decision Making	• Create in each case a collaborative matrix among clinicians involved, patient, and family members • Assessment and diagnostic formulation as dialogal and joint understanding • Shared decision making for clinical care • Conducting health actions with a spirit of shared responsibility
People-Centered Organization of Services	• Identification of community health problems and needs • Planning, development, and implementation of services in collaboration with the community • Establishment of community mechanisms for monitoring and monitoring of services • Integration between health and social services in the community
Person-Centered Education and Research	• Attention to personal development, and not only professional concerns of student, teacher, and researcher • Scientific research of the total person and not only of illness • Consideration of the participation of the person in the different phases of scientific investigations • Strengthening of organizational policies and mechanisms for the cultivation of ethics in educational and research institutions

The principles of person-centered medicine presented in this article are also giving rise to the development of measurement instruments such as the Person-Centered Care Index [23] and its application in the evaluation of person-centered health services [31].

The value of person-centered medicine for substantiating medical education has been a long standing concern of the International College of Person Centered Medicine. This is documented through Declarations emanating from the First and Fourth International Congresses of Person Centered Medicine in Zagreb [32] and in Madrid [33], respectively, and explicated in academic papers accompanying those Declarations [34, 35]. The relevance of person-centered approaches to medical education has wide resonance in the international literature [36]. Furthermore, the Royal College of Psychiatrists in the United Kingdom has pointedly and officially recommended that the professional training of psychiatrists be guided by the values and procedures of person-centered care [37].

In any case, the value of the practical strategies for a person-centered clinical approach proposed in this article must be documented through empirical evaluations. Such studies are recommended both locally and internationally.

CONCLUSIONS

The listed principles and strategies appear promising to clarify both the key concepts of the person-centered medicine movement and to develop useful strategies for clinical care and medical education. By way of synthesis and taking into account the conceptual developments presented in this article and its practical perspectives, it can be said that person-centered medicine proposes clinical care and medical education informed by evidence, experience, and values, and aimed at restoring and promoting the health and well-being of the total person, whatever his or her roles may be.

ACKNOWLEDGMENTS AND DISCLOSURES

The authors report no conflicts of interest.

REFERENCES

1. Heath I. 2005. Promotion of Disease and Corrosion of Medicine. Canadian Family Physician 51: 1320–1322.
2. Miles A. 2009. On a Medicine for the Whole Person: A Way from Scientistic Reductionism and towards the Embrace of Complex Clinical Practice. Journal of Evaluation in Clinical Practice 15: 941–949.
3. Patwardhan B, Warude D, Pushpangadan P, Bhatt N. 2005. Ayurvedic and Traditional Chinese Medicine: A Comparative Overview. Evidence-Based Complementary and Alternative Medicine 2: 465–473.
4. Christodoulou GN (eds). 1987. Psychosomatic Medicine. Plenum Press, New York.
5. Jouanna J. 1999. Hippocrates. Translated by M.B. Debevoise. Johns Hopkins University Press, Baltimore.
6. Anzures y Bolaños MC. 1978. Medicinas tradicionales y antropología. Anales de Antropología (I.I.A./U.N.A.M., México) 15: 151.
7. Mariátegui J. 1992. La concepción del hombre y de la enfermedad en el antiguo Perú. Revista de Neuropsiquiatría 55: 156–166.
8. World Health Organization. 1946. Constitution of the World Health Organization. WHO, Geneva.
9. Delgado H. 1992. El Médico, la Medicina y el Alma. Ediciones Universidad Peruana Cayetano Heredia, Lima.
10. Seguin CA. 1982. La enfermedad, el enfermo y el médico. Ediciones Pirámide, Madrid.
11. Seguín CA. 1993. Tú y la Medicina. Editorial Poniente, Lima.
12. Mezzich JE. 2007. Psychiatry for the Person: Articulating Medicine's Science and Humanism. World Psychiatry 6: 65–67.
13. Mezzich JE. 2010. Repensando el centro de la medicina: De la enfermedad a la persona. Acta Médica Peruana. Versión On-line ISSN 1728–5917.
14. World Health Organization. Resolution on Primary Health Care, Including

Health System Strengthening. In: Sixty-Second World Health Assembly, Geneva, May 18–22, 2009. Resolutions and Decisions. Geneva, 2009 (WHA62/2009/REC/1), page 16.

15. World Health Organization. 2014. Global Strategy for People-Centered Integrated Health Services. World Health Organization, Geneva.

16. Miles A, Mezzich JE. 2011. Advancing the Global Communication of Scholarship and Research for Personalized Healthcare. International Journal of Person Centered Medicine 1: 1–5.

17. Mezzich JE, Botbol M, Christodoulou GN, Cloninger CR, Salloum IM (eds). 2016. Person Centered Psychiatry. Springer, Cham (Switzerland).

18. Wagner P, Perales A, Armas R, Codas O, de los Santos R, Elio-Calvo D, Mendoza-Vega J, Arce M, Calderón JL, Llosa L, Saavedra J, Ugarte O, Vildózola H, Mezzich JE. 2015. Bases y perspectivas latinoamericanas sobre medicina y salud centradas en la pesona. Annales de la Facultad de Medicina (Lima) 76: 63–70.

19. Mezzich JE, Snaedal J, van Weel C, Heath I. 2009. The International Network for Person-Centered Medicine: Background and First Steps. World Med Journal 55: 104–107.

20. Mezzich JE, Snaedal J, vanWeel C, Heath I (eds). 2010. Conceptual Explorations on Person-Centered Medicine. International Journal for Integrated Care 10 (Suppl).

21. Mezzich JE. 2011. The Geneva Conferences and the Emergence of the International Network of Person-Centered Medicine. Journal of Evaluation in Clinical Practice 17: 333–336.

22. Mezzich JE, Kirisici L, Salloum IM. 2014. ICPCM Project on the Systematic Conceptualization and Measurement of Person- and People-Centered Care. Technical Report, International College of Person Centered Medicine, New York.

23. Mezzich JE, Kirisci L, Salloum IM, Adams N, Wallcraft J, Trivedi JK, Kar S K. 2016. Systematically Conceptualizing Person Centered Medicine and Development and Validation of a Measurement Index. International Journal of Person Centered Medicine 16: 219–247.

24. Seguín CA. 2007. El Quinto Oído. Segunda Edición. Instituto Carlos Alberto Seguín, Lima.

25. Leyns C, De Maeseneer J. 2013. Conceptualizing Person- and People-Centeredness in Primary Health Care: A Literature Review. International Journal of Person Centered Medicine 3: 13–22.

26. Harding E. 2016, April 12. Global "State of Play" of Person-Centered Care. Paper presented at the 9th Geneva Conference on Person Centered Medicine, Geneva, Switzerland.

27. Mezzich JE, Salloum IM, Cloninger CR, Salvador-Carulla L, Kirmayer L, Banzato CE, Wallcraft J, Botbol M. 2010. Person-Centered Integrative Diagnosis: Conceptual Bases and Structural Model. Canadian Journal of Psychiatry 55:701–708.
28. Asociación Psiquiátrica de América Latina. 2013. Guía Latinoamericana de Diagnóstico Psiquiátrico, Versión Revisada (GLADP-VR). Sección APAL de Diagnóstico y Clasificación, Lima.
29. Asociación Psiquiátrica de América Latina. 2004. Guía Latinoamericana de Diagnóstico Psiquiátrico, (GLADP). Sección APAL de Diagnóstico y Clasificación, APAL, San Carlos de Sonora, Mexico.
30. Saavedra JE, Mezzich JE, Otero A, Salloum IM. 2012. The Revision of the Latin American Guide for Psychiatric Diagnosis (GLADP) and an Initial Survey on Its Utility and Prospects. International Journal of Person Centered Medicine 2: 214–221.
31. Kirisci L, Hayes J, Mezzich JE. 2016. Evaluation of Person-Centered Health Services. In: Mezzich JE, Botbol M, Christodoulou GN, Cloninger CR, Salloum IM (eds): Person Centered Psychiatry. Springer Verlag, Heidelberg and New York.
32. International College of Person Centered Medicine. 2014. Zagreb Declaration on Person Centered Health Professional Education. International Journal of Person Centered Medicine 4: 6–7.
33. International College of Person Centered Medicine. 2017. Madrid Declaration on Person Centered Medical Education and the Goals of Healthcare. International Journal of Person Centered Medicine 7: 80–81.
34. Appleyard J, Ghebrehiwet T, Mezzich JE. 2014. Development and Implications of the Zagreb Declaration on Person-Centered Health Professional Education. International Journal of Person Centered Medicine 4: 8–13.
35. Appleyard A, Botbol N, Caballero F, Ghebrehiwet T, Mezzich JE, Perez-Miranda J, Ruiz-Moral R, Salloum IM, Snaedal J, Van Leberghe W. 2017. Bases of the Madrid Declaration on Person Centered Medical Education to Enhance Health Systems Worldwide. International Journal of Person Centered Medicine 7 (2): 82–90.
36. Frenk J, Chen L, Butta Z et al. 2010. Health Professionals for a New Century: Transforming Education to Strengthen Health Systems in an Interdependent World. Lancet 376 (9756): 1923–1958.
37. Royal College of Psychiatrists. 2018. Person-Centered Care: Implications for Training in Psychiatry. College Report CR215, London, Author.

MEDICAL PROFESSIONALISM AND ETHICAL AND HUMAN RIGHTS FOUNDATIONS OF PERSON-CENTERED MEDICINE

Jon Snaedal, MD[a]

ABSTRACT

Person-centered medicine (PCM) is a concept that has gained increased acceptance, being a broader term than patient-centered medicine. With PCM the whole of a person is taken into consideration, whether healthy or in disease as well as his or her family. The person of the health professional is also incorporated in this concept. In this article, ethical background to person-centeredness in universal declarations and some international central policies are addressed. Primarily, the UN Universal Declaration on Human Rights (UDHR) will be discussed as well as official policy documents of the World Medical Association (WMA). Lastly, the content of a WMA Declaration on Medical Professionalism are discussed.

Keywords: human rights, health, medical ethics, person-centered medicine, medical professionalism

Correspondence Address: Prof. Jon Snaedal, Ranargata 36, 101 Reykjavik, Iceland.

E-mail: jsnaedal@landspitali.is

INTRODUCTION

Person-centered medicine (PCM) takes into consideration the whole of a person, whether healthy or during disease, as well as his or her family [1]. Using the concept of PCM, two different notions are contradicted. The first model is the classical paternalistic approach toward patients, where patients are at risk of becoming a passive target of therapeutic intervention. In many ways, this has been challenged by increased autonomy of individuals receiving health care and based

---

[a] Professor of Geriatric Medicine, Geriatric Clinic, Landspitali University Hospital, Reykjavik, Iceland; Former President, World Medical Association

on several different processes. One is the model of PCM by which the person/ patient becomes an active collaborator in the patient–physician interaction in several stages such as through the diagnostic process or in therapeutic planning or care, very often of a long-term illness or disability [2]. This has also been reflected in concepts such as "Shared Decision Making" [3]. PCM seems to be more holistic than most other concepts. The other model PCM is contradicting is the organ-specific specialization that has been driven by an immense technical evolution that has led to increased fragmentation of health care. By that the person/patient has become an organ-specific target rather than being considered a whole person [4]. This differs though between different specialization, some being more holistic than others such as primary health care, rehabilitation medicine, psychiatry and geriatric medicine.

One of the hallmarks of the progress medicine has made is the concept of evidence-based medicine (EBM), which has led to a great progress in medical science [5]. This is an approach to medical practice intended to optimize decision making by emphasizing the use of evidence from well-designed and well-conducted research. EBM requires that only the strongest types of research yield strong recommendations such as randomized controlled trials and meta-analysis. Weaker types such as from case-control studies will only lead to weak recommendations [5]. Thus EBM inherently relies primarily on research on groups in contrast to PCM that focuses on the individual person.

PCM must be based on general ethical and human rights and for that some central declarations by international bodies will be reviewed. These are international policies developed by the United Nations (UN), the World Health Organization (WHO), and the World Medical Association (WMA). Lastly, medical professionalism and competence will be addressed using some policies of WMA as background because irrespective of whether we consider PCM or EBM, these fundamental approaches are of profound importance for successful outcome in health care.

THE UN UNIVERSAL DECLARATION ON HUMAN RIGHTS (UDHR) AND THE CONSTITUTION OF WHO

The most widespread foundation of international human rights is the United Nations (UN) Universal Declaration on Human Rights (UDHR). The declaration was one of the first major policies adopted following the establishment of the UN 1945 and is a milestone document in the history of human rights.

The UN General Assembly in Paris proclaimed the Declaration on 10 December 1948 as a common standard of achievements for all peoples and all nations. It sets out, for the first time, fundamental human rights to be universally protected. It contains 30 different paragraphs of which the first sets down the fundament of human rights: *"All human beings are born free and equal in dignity and rights. They are endowed with reason and conscience and should act towards one another in a spirit of brotherhood."*

The original UDHR did not stipulate the right to health or health service in a special article but this is however incorporated in article 25: *"Everyone has the right to a standard of living adequate for the health and well-being of himself and of his family, including food, clothing, housing and medical care and necessary social services, and the right to security in the event of unemployment, sickness, disability, widowhood, old age or other lack of livelihood in circumstances beyond his control."*

It is of interest that the concept well-being is incorporated in this article and it is most likely that this fact is reflecting the influence of the Constitution of the World Health Organization adopted two years earlier. The UDHR has now commemorated its 70th anniversary [6] and to mark its anniversary, a campaign was started to make it better known having high-profile persons to read different paragraphs and posted on social media. The legal significance of the UDHR has been debated, but many argue that due to its general acceptance, it might be legally binding [7]. Legally binding or not, the impact has been immeasurable.

The relationship between human rights and person-centered medicine has been explicated by two former presidents of the WMA, in connection with discussions at a Geneva Conference on Person Centered Medicine [8].

As stated earlier, in 1946 the Constitution of the World Health Organization (WHO) was adopted. In that, the universal definition on health was defined as *"a state of complete physical, mental and social well-being and not merely the absence of disease or infirmity."* The preamble further states *"the enjoyment of the highest attainable standard of health is one of the fundamental rights of every human being without distinction of race, religion, political belief, economic or social condition."* By incorporating well-being, this declaration profoundly altered the concept of health that up till then had considered health as a status of absence of disease [9]. These two internationally adopted principles, the UDHR and the WHO constitution, are therefore in good harmony with each other and inherently person-centered.

THE WORLD MEDICAL ASSOCIATION (WMA)

The World Medical Association (WMA) is representing more than 9 million physicians worldwide. The policies adopted by the WMA have therefore a central role in the physician's everyday work and their ethical conduct. They have also implications for other health professionals, and some of them have gained universal acceptance, mainly the "WMA Declaration of Helsinki on Ethical Principles for Medical Research Involving Human Subjects" [10].

One of the first policies to be adopted by the WMA was the physician's oath or pledge named the Declaration of Geneva (DoG). The horror of World War II was in immediate memory and the newly built international body of physicians felt it necessary to revisit the old Hippocratic oath and to confirm its central content. This pledge was revised in 2017 and is intended to be adopted by medical students at their graduation from medical school and when entering the field of medicine [11].

The International Code of Medical Ethics (ICME) was adopted by WMA in its third General Assembly in 1949. This policy deals in more depth with ethical issues than the DoG and has the form of a declaration rather than a pledge. It addresses in general terms the major ethical challenges a physician faces in their professional life but it also puts some focus on their private life such as the responsibility to attend to own health: "A physician shall seek appropriate care and attention if he/she suffers from mental or physical illness" [12]. The ICME is now undergoing major revision and according to plan, the revision will make use of an open consultation process intended to by finalized in 2021.

Medial professionalism has evolved in many ways; from autonomy to accountability, from expert opinion to evidence-based medicine, from self-interest to teamwork and shared responsibility. The definition of medical professionalism and competence put forward by Epstein and Hundert in 2002 reflects current views [13]: "Professional competence is the habitual and judicious use of communication, knowledge, technical skills, clinical reasoning, emotions, values, and reflection in daily practice for the benefit of the individual and community being served."

In the WMA Declaration of Seoul on Professional Autonomy, reaffirmed in 2018 [14] it states that professional autonomy and clinical independence are core elements of medical professionalism. Furthermore, it is stated that "Professional autonomy and independence are essential for the delivery of high quality health care and therefore benefit patients and society."

Irrespective of how medical professionalism has been considered through the years, it must always be based on the ethical foundation of the medical profession with roots in antiquity. The ethics of doctors involve having human rights as its core element ever more evident with the increasing demand on individual autonomy. However, today, the autonomy of patients is increasingly putting a strain on the ethical values shared by most, as the wishes of patients may be conflicting with those values. WMA laid out the basis for the rights of patients in its Declaration of Lisbon (DoL) [15]. In its preamble it is stated: "while a physician should always act according to his/her conscience, and always in the best interests of the patient, equal effort must be made to guarantee patient autonomy and justice." Rights of patients are described in more detail in the policy containing issues such as the right to medical care of good quality, freedom of choice, self-determination, and dignity as well as the right to religious assistance although that is very different between cultures.

Furthermore, it is stated that physicians and other persons or bodies involved in the provision of health care have a joint responsibility to recognize and uphold these rights. An important way of achieving these goals, shared decision making, is however not addressed in this document.

The importance of medical professionalism is not only its inherent value but it seems as increased nonindependence and lack of professional autonomy is the main cause of increasing burn out of physicians currently reaching epidemic proportions [16]. This is being addressed by the International College of Person Centered Medicine, both in conferences and by adopting Declaration coming out of the discussions in these conferences. For this, the "2019 Geneva Declaration on Person Centered Promotion on Well Being and Overcoming Burn Out" that came from the 12th Geneva Conference on Person Centered Medicine should be kept in mind [17]. Its first recommendation gives the tone: *"The common vision of health care must be person-centered. Organizations of healthcare providers and recipients need to work together to develop and communicate a common vision of the future dedicated with respect for the intrinsic dignity of all people, rather than treating people as dehumanized objects, consumers, or dispensable employees."*

The Declaration continues by recommending that all stakeholders in health care adhere to these principles of person-centeredness in order to promote well-being and overcome burn-out. This has been further developed at the 7th Congress on Person Centered Medicine in Tokyo in November 2019, a collaborative effort by ICPCM and the Japan Medical Association [18].

ACKNOWLEDGMENTS AND DISCLOSURES

The author does not report any conflicts of interest concerning the preparation of this paper.

REFERENCES

1. Mezzich J, Snaedal J, van Weel C, Heath I. 2010. Toward Person-Centered Medicine: From Disease to Patient to Person. Mount Sinai Journal of Medicine 77 (3): 304–306.
2. Leplege A, Gzil F, Cammelin M, Lefeve C, Pachoud D, Cille I. 2007.

Person-Centeredness: Conceptual and Historical Perspectives. Disability and Rehabilitation 29: 1555–1565.

3. Elwyn G, Frosch D, Thomson R, Joseph-Williams N, Lloyd A, Barry M et al. 2012. Shared Decision Making: A Model for Clinical Practice. Journal of General Internal Medicine 27 (10): 1361–1367.

4. Plsek PE, Greenhalgh T. 2001. Complexity Science: The Challenge of Complexity in Health Care. British Medical Journal 323 (7313): 625–628.

5. Eddy DM. 1990. Practice Policies: Where Do They Come from. Journal of the American Medical Association 263 (9): 1265–1272.

6. Brown G. 2016. The Universal Declaration of Human Rights in the 21st Century: A Living Document in a Changing World. Open Book Publishers, United Kingdom. ISBN 978-1-783-74218-9.

7. Steiner HJ, Alston P. 2000. International Human Rights in Context: Law, Politics, Morals, (2nd ed), Oxford University Press, Oxford.

8. Desai K, Appleyard J. 2017. Human Rights and Person Centered Medicine: The Need of the Hour. International Journal of Person Centered Medicine 7 (3): 161–164.

9. Grad FP. 2002. The Preamble of the Constitution of the World Health Organization. Bulletin of the World Health Organization 80 (12): 981–982.

10. The World Medical Declaration of Helsinki on Ethical Principles for Medical Research Involving Human Subjects. Journal of the American Medical Association 310 (29): 2191–2194.

11. https://www.wma.net/policies-post/wma-declaration-of-geneva

12. https://www.wma.net/policies-post/wma-international-code-of-medical-ethics

13. Epstein RM, Hundert EM. 2002. Defining and Assessing Professional Competence. Journal of the American Medical Association 287 (2): 226–235.

14. https://www.wma.net/policies-post/wma-declaration-of-seoul-on-professional-autonomy-and-clinical-independence

15. https://www.wma.net/policies-post/wma-declaration-of-lisbon-on-the-rights-of-the-patient

16. Rothenberger DA. 2017. Physician Burnout and Well-Being: A Systematic Review and Framework for Action. Diseases of the Colon & Rectum 60 (6): 567–576.

17. https://www.personcenteredmedicine.org/doc/2019-pdf/04/2019-Geneva-Declaration.pdf

18. https://www.personcenteredmedicine.org/doc/2019-pdf/Tokyo-International-Congress.pdf

THE MAKING OF A PHYSICIAN:
A PERSON-CENTERED APPROACH

Shridhar Sharma, MD, FRCPsy(Lond), DPM, FRANZCP(Aus),
DFAPA(USA), FAMS[a] and Gautam Sharma, MD[b]

ABSTRACT

The subject "The Making of a Physician: A Person-Centered Approach" is important today because of the current changing health care environment, where the practice of medicine is being increasingly influenced by growth in science, technology, high cost, rising expectations of the people, and other powerful market forces emerging from the globalization process, which have put medical practice at cross roads.

The essence of medicine lies in the therapeutic relationship between the doctor and the patient and our attitude to our patients.

It is the person in totality that we are interested in both in health and disease. In reality, the relief of suffering and the cure of a person must be seen as twin obligations of the profession, and true dedication to the cure of the sick. The cure of disease is influenced by our scientific knowledge and growth of science, while the relief of suffering is guided by our compassion to the patient and sharing of patients' suffering and feelings.

Keywords: making of physician, medical practice, person-centered medicine, humanism, ethics, medical education

Correspondence Address: Prof. Shridhar Sharma, D-127, Preet Vihar, Vikas Marg, Delhi – 110092, India

E-mail: Sharma.shridhar@gmail.com

INTRODUCTION

Humanism and science are intimately linked and have a dynamic relationship. In the context of the scientific paradigm, the essential misses much of the essence of medical practice, which should be person- and not disease-centered. It is the

---

[a] Emeritus Professor, National Academy of Medical Sciences & Institute of Human Behaviour and Allied Sciences, New Delhi, India
[b] Associate Professor, Department of Psychiatry, R.M.L. Hospital, New Delhi, India

person in totality that we are interested in both health and disease. It was Hippocrates [1], who had aptly remarked "I would rather know the person who has the disease than know the disease the person has." Later in the early twentieth century Rudolf Virchow [2], an eminent German pathologist, had reiterated that "The proper objects are not diseases but conditions in a person." Today we are forgetting the person but treating only the disease. In reality, the relief of suffering and the cure of a person must be seen as twin obligations of the profession, and true dedication to the cure of the sick. The cure of disease is influenced by our scientific knowledge and growth of technology, while the relief of suffering is guided by our compassion and our ability to communicate with the patient [3].

Technology certainly provides new tools for clinicians in the field of diagnosis, treatment, and in aiding disability and "New Hopes for the Patients." However, irrational diffusion of technology has negative consequences. It is also necessary to carefully examine the related cost-benefit of treatment and ethical questions. To grasp these aspects, it is essential to continuously assess growth of cost-effective technology and its appropriate use in the health field. Science can be just as potent for good as for evil.

"It is not science, however which will determine how science is used. Science by itself cannot supply an ethics. It can show us how to achieve a given end and it may show us that some ends cannot be achieved. But among ends that can be achieved, our choice must be decided by other than purely scientific consideration." Humanism and science are intimately linked and have a dynamic relationship. It seems obvious to many in the profession of medicine that in the context of the scientific paradigm of today, the essential misses much of the essence of medical practice [4, 5]. To support this view, many authors have emphasized that modern medicine must emphasize the humane and compassionate aspects of medicine. If taught properly with quality and sensitivity, principles of humanism should be a necessary and continuing reminder to all in medicine of its mission. But what the humane and compassionate aspects of medicine are and what defines quality and sensitivity is not made clear.

CORE PROFESSIONAL VALUES

The value of human life is to be respected whether they are from developed or developing countries. The final answer lies in the conscience of the doctor, a universal respect for human values, and the ideology of humanism. Hence the applications of the basic principles of medical ethics are never static but are continuously evolving to meet ever-changing needs of a society. These issues should not only be plastic but also sensitive to meet the changing needs of social evolution brought out as a result of constant scientific and technological development, the changing sociopolitical ideology, high cost of treatment, rising expectations of the people, and various market forces all of which as powerful actors have put medical practice at a cross roads once again.

These values and determinants related to ethics germinated in almost all ancient civilizations. Many have been confided since the time of Hippocrates. As a continuum of Hippocratic tradition for centuries, physicians had approached the patient from position of paternalism. An individual just because of being in need of medical intervention became ipso facto a patient, a passive being who would be expected to abrogate personal rights as an autonomous person, dependent on decision of the pater-physician, whose decisions were final on issues of treatment and all related circumstances. The patient had no say, into the decisions or the proposed potential solutions. Neither did the physicians have to give any explanations about the diagnosis nor the treatment. The Hippocratic oath imposes on physicians, a duty to secrecy of knowledge and advised secrecy of procedures, without saying anything to patient. The physician was also the confident and the guardian of the secrets of the patient. In return for this power it was expected that physician would neither compromise nor take advantage of his unique position and never to compromise his as a physician or that of his profession to respect the intrinsic values of human life. These values have been subjected to serious pressures and stood the test of time with few exceptions.

A careful review, of all these ethical guidelines and human values, reveal some of the commonalties in all declarations on ethics with relative degree of emphasis on some values. Ethical issues in medicine require a physician to place the human values of patients above all other considerations. It is the basic obligation of each clinician to give his patient the best therapy available at the time. The therapy available at the time may not be applicable to the future or in a different place or situation. The ideal therapy is the therapy with the highest, most specific, and speediest efficacy with the least side effects, risks, or disadvantages to the patient. Hence the applications of the principles in medical ethics are never static. They are continuously evolving to meet the ever-changing needs of a society. These issues should not only be plastic but also sensitive to meet the changing needs of social evolution brought out as a result of constant scientific and technological development and changing sociopolitical ideology, high cost of treatment, rising expectations of the people, and various market forces as powerful actors, all of which have put medical practice at a cross roads once again.

As medicine has become more powerfully scientific, it has also become increasingly depersonalized, so that in some areas of clinical practice an overreliance on science in the care of patients has led to the substitution of scientific medicine with and an accompanying collapse of humanistic value in the profession of medicine. Since medicine has a unalterable imperative to care, comfort, and console as well as to ameliorate, attenuate, and cure, the perpetuation of a modern myth in medicine – that now we can cure we have no more responsibility to care – risks the creation of an ethical and moral chaos within clinical practice and the generation of negative outcomes for both patients and clinicians alike. With reference to these observations and concerns, we briefly review signal occurrences in the development of the so-called "patient as a person" movement.

Learning and updating the science is an essential part of medical profession but it is not always its essence [6]. The essence includes the qualities of humanism, compassion, and empathy to our patients. There is no such thing as valueless medicine. All of us, as we practice, carry our values, professional standards, aims, and goals from the rest of life into our medical practice and much more to the point, and so do our patients, whom doctors care and cure.

PERSON-CENTERED THERAPEUTIC RELATIONSHIP

There is no denying the fact that all the relevant technology and scientific values are essential parts in medicine; the essence of medicine lies in the therapeutic relationship between the doctor and the patient and our attitude, compassion, and empathy to our patients [7]. It is the basic obligation of each clinician, to give his patient the best therapy available at the time at a given place. The therapy available at the time may not be applicable to the future or in a different place or situation. The ideal therapy is the therapy with the highest, most specific, and speediest efficacy with the least side effects, risks, or disadvantages to the patient. One of the reasons for such failure could be due to lack of training received by today's doctors. It is an essential requirement to orient and expose to such sensitive elements during the training process for the making a good physician. The training should also emphasize moral and ethical values and its focus should be person-centered.

A person-centered approach is also important because of the current changing health care environment, where the practice of medicine is being increasingly influenced by growth in science, technology, high costs, and other powerful market forces emerging from the globalization process [8], which have put medical practice at a cross roads. The need for introspection and desirable change arises from a variety of factors and the ramifications of these influences are manifold.

The subject is related to, and dependent on, a large complex of other disciplines belonging to biological sciences, socioeconomic factors, and ethical issues. The relief of suffering and cure of disease are the main objectives of medicine. It is the person in totality that we are interested in both in health and disease. Such a concept requires a rejection of the historical dualism of body and mind. The mind–body dichotomy has resulted in assigning the body to medicine and the person to something else, the mind [9].

The suffering resulting from the pathology of the mind can be to some extent assessed and treated, but suffering resulting from defacement of values and principles is more complex and complicated to manage. Dr. William Osler [9], father of modern medicine, had stated that "medicine is both science and art." Earlier it was presumed that physician was not only a healer but also a custodian and the guardian of the secrets of the patient. In return for this power over the patient, the physician would undertake not to take advantage of the relative weakness of the patient and never to compromise his honor or that of his profession. He was also expected to respect the intrinsic value of human life.

THE ROLE OF PHYSICIANS AND THEIR EDUCATION

Traditionally physicians were not greedy, but their basic needs of living were looked after by the society. He was not only respected but was held in high esteem and which was next to "God." The scientific advances in medicine, concomitant with globalization process, have presented us with extraordinary and unforeseen ethical dilemmas, posing problems that have ramifications far beyond medicine, to society and profession as a whole. Globalization is a system, dictated by an ideology. The ideology is that of "market force economics," where the invisible hand of the market mechanism is allowed to operate unimpeded in a globalized world.

There is no such thing as valueless medicine. All of us, as we practice medicine, carry our values, professional standards, aims, and goals from the rest of life into our medical practice, and so do our patients, whom doctors care and cure. The twentieth-century Canadian physician and father of modern medicine, Sir William Osler, composed a famous essay on the importance of equanimity when practicing medicine [10].

Though there is some awareness on this aspect during training program in medicine but the fact remains that there is obvious lack of stress on such elements in the training program. On the other hand, the scientific content of training is increasingly technology oriented, which is essential, but the essence of medicine is missing. The need to incorporate "value" and "compassion" in care to our patients, in the schematization of training program and later integrating in daily medical practice, is very urgent. An ethical and value-based approach must be regarded as a part of the therapeutic effort in any management endeavor.

There is an urgent need to introduce these elements in training programs in the making of a doctor. This aspect of training is vital for effective professional functioning and the growth of the medical profession as a discipline and within a specialty, which is respected and held in high esteem. It is the responsibility of the senior professionals in the field of medicine, to play an important role, as an advocate for the humanitarian principles of medicine and also help in shaping medicine as a valued profession in a changing materialistic environment.

CONCLUSION

What is required is the commitment of medical professionals to the profession, with qualities of compassion and sensitivity and to appreciate, feel, and understand some of the fading qualities and values of the practice of medicine. There is an old saying "who is not a good man shall not make a good physician" [11] and "one cannot help the patient without understanding the man." [12]

ACKNOWLEDGMENTS AND DISCLOSURES

The authors do not report any conflicts of interest concerning this paper.

REFERENCES

1. William VW. 2012. Book Review: Hippocrates Is Not Dead: An Anthology of Hippocratic Readings. By Guinan P. Linacre Q. 79(3): 370–373. Doi 10.1179/002436312804872776 PMCID: PMC6027038
2. Virchow R. 1989. The Huxley Lecture on Recent Advances in Science and their Bearing on Medicine and Surgery: Delivered at the opening of the Charing Cross Hospital Medical School. British Medical Journal 2 (1971): 1021–1028.
3. Miles A. 2009. Towards a Medicine of the Whole Person: Knowledge, Practice and Holism in the Care of the Sick. Journal of Evaluation in Clinical Practice 15: 887–890.
4. Mezzich JE, Snaedal J, van Weel C, Heath I. 2010. From Disease to Patient to Person: Towards a Person-Centered Medicine. Mount Sinai Journal of Medicine 77: 304–306.
5. Mezzich JE, Snaedal J, van Weel C, Botbol M, Salloum I. 2011. Introduction to Person-Centered Medicine: From Concepts to Practice. Journal of Evaluation in Clinical Practice 17: 330–332.
6. Miles A, Mezzich JE. 2011. The Care of the Patient and the Soul of the Clinic: Person-Centered Medicine as an Emergent Model of Modern Clinical Practice. International Journal of Person Centered Medicine 1 (2): 207–222. DOI: 10.5750/ijpcm.v1i2.617.

7. Borrell-Carrio F, Suchman AL, Epstein RM. 2004. The Biopsychosocial Model 25 Years later: Principles, Practice and Scientific Inquiry. Annals of Family Medicine 2: 576–582.
8. Woodward J, Drager N, Beaglehole R, Lipson D. 2001. Globalization and Health, a Frame Work for Analysis and Action. Bulletin of the World Health Organization 79: 875–881.
9. William Osler. https://en.wikipedia.org/wiki/William_Osler10.
10. Gryglewski Ryszard J. 1995. Medicine: How Much Science, How Much Art, Jagiellonian Medical Research Centre, Cracow, Poland, pp. v–vi.
11. Biegański W. 1908. Logika medycyny czyli krytyka poznania lekarskiego, wyd. 2 na nowo oprac. Warszawa: E. Wende i S-ka.
12. Aleksandrowicz J. 1985. Studia meaticzne a etos zawodu lekarza A.M. Krakow.

CONCEPTS AND STRATEGIES OF PEOPLE-CENTERED PUBLIC HEALTH

Fredy A. Canchihuaman, MD, MPH, PhD[a], W. James Appleyard, MA, MD, FRCP[b], and Juan E. Mezzich, MD, MA, MSc, PhD[c]

ABSTRACT

Introduction: Public health is a discipline that focuses on populations and aims to prevent, promote, and protect health and well-being of individuals and communities. Different factors have limited the effectiveness of public health to achieve their goals. New perspectives to strengthen public health have been recommended.

Objective: To examine and describe concepts and strategies of people-centered public health.

Methods: A review of the scientific literature was conducted to delineate the links between public health and the person-centered approach. In order to refine the core elements of a person-centered approach suitable for public health, the International College of Person Centered Medicine's "Person-Centered Care Index" was adapted using as reference guidelines containing principles for public health practice.

Results: Modern public health has been strengthened by the influence of various strategies and approaches such as the determinants of health, Universal Health Coverage, Primary Health Care, noncommunicable diseases actions, and Sustainable Development Goals. Public health could further be strengthened by the influence of the people-centered approach. This approach reflects adherence to fundamental human, medical, and public ethics principles and values and a holistic conception of persons with spiritual, biological, social, cultural, and psychological elements. Hence, people-centered public health in practice denotes

[a] Professor of Public Health, Universidad Peruana Cayetano Heredia, Lima, Peru

[b] Board Advisor and Former President, International College of Person Centered Medicine; Former President, World Medical Association; Former President, International Association of Medical Colleges

[c] Professor of Psychiatry, Icahn School of Medicine at Mount Sinai, New York; Hipólito Unanue Chair of Person Centered Medicine, San Fernando Medical School, San Marcos National University, Lima, Peru; Former President, World Psychiatric Association; Former President and current Secretary General, International College of Person Centered Medicine

public health activities and functions guided by these principles, values, and concepts. The core elements of the people-centered public health approach (person-centered approach relevant to public health) based on the "Person-Centered Care Index" are (1) Ethical Commitment, (2) Cultural Awareness and Responsiveness, (3) Holistic Approach, (4) Relational Focus, (5) Individualization of Care, (6) Common Ground for Collaborative Actions and Shared Decision Making, (7) People-Centered Organization of Systems, and (8) Evidence Informed and Persons-Centered Education and Research. A key feature of the people-centered public health approach is the articulation of public health and clinical care and of person- and people-centered approaches.

Conclusions: Adopting a people-centered public health approach may critically enhance population health and contribute to international efforts toward achieving Universal Health Coverage and Sustainable Development Goals.

Keywords: person- and people-centered approach, public health, health systems, improving population health, ethics, holistic approach, cultural awareness and responsiveness, relational focus, individualized care, common grounds for collaborative actions, persons-centered public health, evidence-informed and person-centered education and research.

Correspondence Address: Dr. Fredy Canchihuaman, Facultad de Salud Pública y Administración, Universidad Peruana Cayetano Heredia, Avenida Honorio Delgado 430, Lima 31, Perú.

E-mail: canchihuaman.fredy@gmail.com

THE SCOPE OF PUBLIC HEALTH

Charles Edward Winslow back in 1920 defined public health as "the science and the art of preventing disease, prolonging life, and promoting physical health and efficiency through organized community efforts" [1]. This new definition, based on reflections about its future evolution, was a breakthrough in the development of this field. Currently, this description of public health with minimal changes remains tentatively valid and accepted even though there is not a wide consensus [2].

Public Health Functions

Public health is an evolving discipline and has been influenced historically and recently by strategies and approaches such as the Determinants of Health, Primary

Health Care, Noncommunicable Diseases Actions, Health Promotion, Universal Health Coverage, and the Sustainable Development Goals [3, 4]. Activities and services related to public health have been grouped in a number of core functions called "essential public health functions"; a concept that varies among organizations and countries [2, 5] (see Table 1).

Table 1. Essential Public Health Functions from International Organizations

Essential Public Health Functions, CDC, CLAISS, and PAHO (American Region, 2001)	Essential Public Health Operations, WHO (European Region, 2007–2014)	Essential Public Health Services, CDC (USA, 1994)
1. Health situation monitoring and analysis 2. Surveillance, research, and control of the risks and threats to public health 3. Health promotion 4. Social participation in health 5. Development of policies and institutional capacity for public health planning and management 6. Strengthening of public health regulation and enforcement capacity 7. Evaluation and promotion of equitable access to necessary health services 8. Human resources development and training in public health 9. Quality assurance in personal- and population-based health services 10. Research in public health 11. Reduction of the impact of emergencies and disasters on health	1. Monitoring, evaluation, and analysis of health status 2. Monitoring and response to health hazards and emergencies 3. Health protection, including environmental, occupational, food safety, and others 4. Health promotion, including action to address social determinants and health inequity 5. Disease prevention, including early detection of illness 6. Governance for health and well-being 7. Sufficient and competent public health workforce 8. Sustainable organizational structures and financing 9. Information, communication, and social mobilization for health 10. Public health research to inform policy and practice	1. Monitoring, evaluation, and analysis of health status 2. Diagnosing and investigating health problems and health hazards in the community 3. Informing, educating, and empowering people about health issues 4. Mobilizing community partnerships to identify and solve health problems 5. Developing policies and plans that support individual and community health efforts 6. Enforcing laws and regulations that protect health and ensure safety 7. Linking people to needed personal health services and assuring the provision of health care when otherwise unavailable 8. Assuring a competent public and personal health care workforce 9. Evaluating effectiveness, accessibility, and quality of personal- and population-based health services 10. Searching for new insights and innovative solutions to health problems

Taken from: World Health Organization. Essential Public Health Functions, Health Systems and Health Security: Developing Conceptual Clarity and a WHO Roadmap for Action. World Health Organization; 2018 [5].

Challenges of Public Health

There are several problems that limit modern public health to effectively undertake their functions and achieve their goals. Inadequate organizational structure and capacity to address public health threats, constrained scope of action, insufficient allocated resources, and predominant biomedical approaches to health, among others, has been reported [6, 7]. These problems related to public health occur globally, even in developed countries. A disordered organizational structure of public health has been considered itself as a public health threat; since only effective collective actions – public health actions – might secure proper health conditions and prevent, control, and resolve sustained and emergent threats at the population level [7]. Recent events within the infection disease arena such as infection diseases outbreaks have illustrated the inadequate capacity to collectively address these kinds of threats to global public health [8].

The Individual and Its Context

The wide conception of health – that considers that health and well-being of a person is also determined by their context – is the foundation of approaches, models, and strategies focusing on the health at the community level [9].

Public health approaches addressing health at the group or community level might vary. The population health approach, proposed by the Public Health Agency of Canada [10], considers, for example, eight elements with its corresponding actions that define this particular approach: "focus on the health of populations; address the determinants of health and their interactions; base decisions on evidence; increase upstream investments; apply multiple strategies; collaborate across sectors and levels; employ mechanisms for public involvement; and demonstrate accountability for health outcomes." The population health approach is described by other authors as the "wide range of factors and interrelated conditions that influence the health of populations over the life course, identifies systematic variations in their patterns of occurrence, and applies the resulting knowledge to improve the health and well-being of those populations" [11, 12]. Both share in common a people dimension rather than individual while undertaking actions on health issues.

Although, public health implies focuses on group health, some authors have claimed that population health is a wider approach than public health [11]; given the fact that public health out into the real practice has a restrained field of action and does not necessarily address various determinants of health. These and other factors have motivated some authors to propose new public health models, as the public health 3.0, to move outside the traditional public health practices [13].

47

To consolidate the advancement of public health worldwide, it is necessary to embrace a wider and holistic approach to public health; and a people-centered public health approach might address this requirement.

A WAY FORWARD: IMPROVING POPULATION HEALTH

The person-centered approach is founded in the recognition that the rights of both liberty and welfare are essential [14]. This means that it puts an equivalent value to the liberty of a person as well as the responsibility of a person to the welfare of others and the environment [14, 15]. This approach implies a natural commitment to principles and values of "equity, social justice, sustainable development (...) and those of medical ethics" [6] and to a holist conception of persons with its different elements spiritual, biological, social, cultural, and psychological [15]. The person-centered approach has also itself been considered as an "ethical mandate" [16]. In consequence, this approach, what it encourages is a medical practice guided by these principles, values, and concepts. Furthermore, it has been suggested that both clinical health and public health practices "should share these values" [6].

In the case of public health, a shift to a people-centered public health approach will mean that these principles, values, and concepts are borne in mind while performing public health activities and functions. Though, some additional considerations need to be taken due to the unique character of the public health field; and consequently the medical principles, values, and concepts described previously should be adapted within any analysis of complex public health issues [17]. The ethical principles, values, and concepts of public health ethics field involved in the current discussions are about "relational autonomy" and "community consent," "community beneficence,, "avoidance of harm through collective actions," "group and individual social justice," "health equity," "right to health," "solidarity," "reciprocity," "utility," and "transparency" [17]. Likewise, "public justification" and "fair process" are highlighted as ethical consideration for public health decision making [17, 18].

Elements of the People-Centered Public Health Approach

A comprehensive study on the conceptualization of person-centered approach identified eight distinctive domains as elements converging on this concept [15]. The study consisted of systematic literature reviews and iterative consultation with experts on the core elements of "person-centered medicine, person-centered health care, and person- and people-centered health systems." Initially 14 elements of "Personal Health and Care" and 7 elements of "Public Health and Services

Organization" were identified. A further operationalization of the concepts was performed, which led to the design of a "Person-Centered Care Index" [15].

Since the main focus of the index is on clinical practice, a brief adaptation of these elements relevant to public health practice resulted in the following: (1) Ethical Commitment, (2) Cultural Awareness and Responsiveness, (3) Holistic Approach, (4) Relational Focus, (5) Individualization of Care, (6) Common Ground for Collaborative Actions and Shared Decision Making, (7) People-Centered Organization of Systems, and (8) Evidence Informed and Persons-Centered Education and Research. The adaptation consisted of reviewing guidelines for public health practice; analyzing the content and applicability; and reorganizing and extending the elements with small text edits focusing in populations and around concepts and functions of public health. The following sources were selected for this purpose: the WHO-integrated evidence to decision framework [19], the Principles of the Ethical Practice of Public Health [20], the Public Health Ethics: Cases Spanning the Globe [17], and the PAHO conceptual document on Bioethics: Toward the Integration of Ethics in Health [18] (see Table 2).

Public Health Actions Influenced by the People-Centered Approach

People-centered approach to public health could lead to more efficient public health actions (e.g., enhancing prevention, promotion, protection and prolonging life and addressing social and environmental determinants) and to improvement in the "organization of community efforts" (e.g., developing sustained, continuous and integrated actions throughout the different stages of people lives, and promoting articulation of public health and primary care, universal health, and sustainable development). While in the medical and research field guiding principles are prolific for practice, this is not the case in the public health field despite of the significant impact of public health practice in many people's lives. The core elements of the people-centered public health approach might help to reorient public health functions, decisions, and actions and guide the path toward a public health for all (see Table 2).

Integration of Public Health and Primary Care: A Key Strategy for People-Centered Public Health

A particular feature of the people-centered public health approach deriving from at least two of its elements ("community-based systems of care" and "holistic scope") is the advocacy for an integration of public health and clinical care [6].

Evidence suggests that the integration of public health and primary care might be more effective to improve community health, well-being [21], and resources

49

Table 2. Elements of Person-Centered and People-Centered Public Health Approaches

Person-Centered Approach [15]	People-Centered Public Health Approach	The WHO-INTEGRATE Evidence to Decision Framework Version 1.0 [19]	Principles of the Ethical Practice of Public Health [20]
Ethical commitment The dignity of every person involved (patients, family, clinicians) is honored Patient's rights are respected Patient's autonomy is supported Patient's empowerment is advanced The fulfillment of the patient's life project (purpose in life) is enabled and encouraged The patient's personal values, choices, and needs are understood and respected	**Ethical commitment** Public health actions and functions' performance should be ethical and based on fundamental human values and principles Public health actions and functions' performance should consider medical and public health ethics perspectives <u>Equity</u> <u>Autonomy</u> <u>Well-being</u> <u>Social justice</u> <u>Solidarity</u> <u>Human rights</u> <u>Right to health</u> <u>Peace</u> <u>Sustainable development</u>	**Balance of health benefits and harms** The balance of health **benefits and harms** reflects the magnitude and types of health impact of an intervention on individuals or populations. **Health equity, equality, and nondiscrimination** Health equity and equality reflect a concerted and sustained effort to improve health for individuals across all populations, and to reduce avoidable systematic differences in how health and its determinants are distributed. Equality is linked to the legal principle of nondiscrimination, which is designed to ensure that individuals or population groups do not experience discrimination on the basis of their sex, age, ethnicity, culture or language, sexual orientation or gender identity, disability status, education, socioeconomic status, place of residence, or any other characteristics.	Public health should achieve community health in a way that **respects the rights** of individuals in the community. Public health institutions should protect the **confidentiality of information** that can bring harm to an individual or community if made public. Exceptions must be justified on the basis of the high likelihood of significant harm to the individual or others.

Table 2. (*Continued*)

Person-Centered Approach [15]	People-Centered Public Health Approach	The WHO-INTEGRATE Evidence to Decision Framework Version 1.0 [19]	Principles of the Ethical Practice of Public Health [20]
Cultural sensitivity The patient's ethnic identity and cultural values are recognized The patient's language and communication needs and preferences are actively considered The patient's gender and sexual preferences are acknowledged and respected The patient's spiritual needs are factored in	**Cultural awareness and responsiveness** Public health actions and functions' performance should be aware and responsive to cultural context; recognizing ethnic identity and cultural values; actively considering language and communication needs and preferences; acknowledging and respecting gender and sexual preferences; and considering the spiritual needs	**Human rights and sociocultural acceptability** Human rights refer to an intervention's compliance with **universal human rights** standards and other considerations laid out in international human rights law beyond the right to health (as the right to health provides the basis of other criteria and subcriteria in this framework). **Sociocultural acceptability** is highly time-specific and context-specific and reflects the extent to which those implementing or benefiting from an intervention as well as other relevant stakeholder groups consider it to be appropriate, based on anticipated or experienced cognitive and emotional responses to the intervention.	Public health programs and policies should incorporate a variety of approaches that anticipate and **respect diverse values, beliefs, and cultures** in the community.

Holistic scope The biological, psychological, social, cultural, and spiritual factors of health inform understanding and care Both ill-health (health problems, disabilities) and positive health or well-being (functioning, resilience, strengths, resources, and quality of life) are focus of attention	**Holistic approach** Public health actions and functions' performance should have a holistic scope; being informed by the biological, psychological, social, cultural, and spiritual factors of community health Public health actions and functions' performance focus of attention should be both ill-health and positive health or well-being Public health actions and functions' performance should be oriented to consider the determinants of health at different levels and to secure access to every person in the community	**Societal implications** Societal implications recognize that health interventions do not take place in isolation and may enhance or inhibit broader **social, environmental, or economic goals** in the short or long term. It also reflects the fact that many regulatory, environmental, or other **population-level health interventions are directly aimed at system-level** rather than individual-level changes.	Public health programs and policies should be implemented in a manner that most **enhances the physical and social environment.** Public health should **address** principally the fundamental **causes of disease and requirements for health,** aiming to **prevent adverse health outcomes.** Public health should advocate for, or work for the empowerment of, disenfranchised community members, ensuring that the basic resources and **conditions necessary for health are accessible to all** people in the community.
Relational focus Clinicians, patients, and families work in partnership Empathy in clinical communication is emphasized Interpersonal trust is fostered throughout the care process	**Relational focus** Public health actions and functions' performance should be a consequence of communication, collaborations, and coordination among different stakeholders at all levels. Promoting partnerships between health care professionals, persons, families, and communities; between health care professionals, health-related professionals, and professional from other disciplines; between primary care and public health providers, managers, and public health authorities; and between programs and health-related sectors. Emphasized empathy in communication and interpersonal and community trust should be fostered throughout the care process.		

Table 2. (*Continued*)

Person-Centered Approach [15]	People-Centered Public Health Approach	The WHO-INTEGRATE Evidence to Decision Framework Version 1.0 [19]	Principles of the Ethical Practice of Public Health [20]
Individualized care The patient's individuality and unique qualities inform care. The patient's historical and social context are factored in The patient's personal growth and development are promoted.	**Individualization of care** Public health actions and functions' performance should be oriented to the communities; informed by the community individuality and unique qualities. Historical and social context of community should be considered Public health actions and functions' performance should promote community growth and development. Actions should be responsive to specific community needs and expectations and be personalized with high quality and excellence		
Common ground for collaborative diagnosis and care Diagnosis of health status, experience, and contributory factors involve shared understanding Diagnosis is worked out taking into account the whole person Care plan decisions are made collaboratively	**Common ground for collaborative actions and shared decision making** Public health actions and functions' performance should be made collaborative and planed, developed and implemented through processes that involve shared understanding and take into account the community as a whole Public health actions and functions' performance should include community participation.		Public health institutions and their employees should engage in **collaborations and affiliations** in ways that build the public's trust and the institution's effectiveness. Public health policies, programs, and priorities should be developed and evaluated through processes that ensure an opportunity for **input from community members.** Public health institutions should **provide communities with the information** they have that is **needed for decisions** on policies or programs and should **obtain the community's consent for** their implementation.

People-centered systems of care	People-centered organization of systems	Feasibility and health system considerations	Public health institutions should ensure the professional competence of their employees.
The health and rights of all people in the community are advocated and promoted The community participates in the planning of health services Collaboration across disciplines and programs is promoted at all levels of service organization Personalized services are aimed at attaining high quality and excellence. Health services are responsive to specific community needs and expectations Health services are integrated and coordinated around patients' needs Services emphasize people-centered primary care Services ensure continuity of care Services are informed by person-centered international perspectives and developments	Public health actions and functions' performance should be system of care oriented. Public health actions and functions' performance should be adapted taking into account the particular characteristics and complexity of health system (in terms of legislation, governance, financing, services organization, and so forth) and the people-centered international perspectives and developments Public health actions and functions' performance should be undertake acknowledging the importance for having an integral, integrated, continuity, and sustained care focusing around persons' needs and expectations. Public health actions and functions' performance should emphasize people-centered primary health care	Feasibility and health system considerations recognize that the most appropriate and feasible interventions may vary significantly across different contexts, both across countries and across jurisdictions within countries. Legislation and governance, the structure of the health system and existing programs, as well as human resources and infrastructure, should be taken into account. **Financial and economic considerations** Financial and economic considerations acknowledge that available financial (budgetary) resources are constrained and take into account the economic impact of an intervention on the health system, government, or society as a whole.	
Person-centered education and research The health system promotes person-centered public education The health system promotes person-centered health professional training The health system promotes person-centered clinical research	**Evidence informed and persons-centered education and research** Public health actions and functions' performance should be pertinent to the context and informed by the best evidence available, experiences, values, and culture	**Quality of evidence** Quality of evidence, also referred to as certainty of evidence or strength of evidence, reflects the confidence that the available evidence is adequate to support a recommendation.	Public health should seek the information needed to implement effective policies and programs that protect and promote health. Public health institutions should act in a timely manner on the information they have within the resources and the mandate given to them by the public.

use [12]. It is more likely to achieve public health and clinical care goals if their actions are performed jointly and complementarily rather than separately and in isolation [6]. On the clinical practice side, integration, meaning clinical practice performed with a public health perspective, might potentially result in individual care with a direct impact on the care of the individual's family and community [6].

A literature review on the role of integration on health systems describes the lack of this as one of the prevailing problems for health systems. The health systems emphasis is on care specialization and illnesses as opposed to better health prevention and promotion through public health and primary health care [22]. This review suggests that in order to create better health systems ("effective, equitable, efficient, [sustainable, universal] and affordable") it is critical the integration of health care, public health and primary health care; which is defined as "health or medical care that begins at time of first contact" with a "societal perspective" and community-based participation. On the other hand, this review also emphasizes the "social-ecological model" as a suitable model to appreciate the relationships and interconnections between individuals, communities, and the society as a whole and to analyze the elements of the health systems (public health, primary health care, and others).

But the term "integration" could be understood differently in different settings. A variety of forms of integration have been identified such as "organizational, functional services, clinical, normative, and systemic" [12]. From this perspective, a comprehensive type of integration has been proposed that merges health care with the "population health approach." For that reason, it is asserted that the integration only of the health services is not sufficient to reach population's health goals and that operational strategies to make comprehensive integration real are urgently needed [12].

MEASURING PERFORMANCE ON PEOPLE-CENTERED PUBLIC HEALTH APPROACH

It is fundamental that public health practice and exercise of public health functions at the different levels within and beyond health systems be conducted following the core elements of people-centered approach. Instruments to measure public health actions might help to provide evidence so that theory is translated into real-world practice. The Person-Centered Care Index is a practical validated tool to measures the absence, presence, and frequency of a set of person-centered activities carried out in health care services [15]. The index has in total 33 variables; each can be rated on a 4-point scale and the set of variables summarized with a global average score. Given its clinical practice orientation, an adapted version of the Person-Centered Care Index is needed for assessing public health practice.

CONCLUSIONS

A people-centered public health approach, as is the case with primary health care [23] and human security [24], could be considered as an underlying philosophy and a general strategy to guide public health policies, public health programs, and public health practices as well as the basis for measuring public health functions' performance. From a practical perspective, the reflection on person or people per se unleashed an instinctive transforming action (e.g., integral care). Adopting a people-centered public health approach may critically enhance population health and contribute to international efforts toward achieving Universal Health Coverage and Sustainable Development Goals.

ACKNOWLEDGMENTS AND DISCLOSURES

The authors report no conflicts of interest in the preparation of this paper.

REFERENCES

1. Winslow CE. 1920. The Untilled Fields of Public Health. Science 51 (1306): 23–33.
2. Rechel B, McKee M, European Observatory on Health Systems and Policies, editors. 2014. Facets of Public Health in Europe. Maidenhead, Berkshire, England: McGraw Hill Education, Open University Press. 346 p. (European Observatory on Health Systems and Policies series).
3. Schmidt H, Gostin LO, Emanuel EJ. 2015. Public Health, Universal Health Coverage, and Sustainable Development Goals: Can They Coexist? Lancet 386 (9996): 928–930.
4. Atrash K, Carpentier R. 2012. The Evolving Role of Public Health in the Delivery of Health Care. Journal of Human Growth and Development 22 (3): 396–399.
5. World Health Organization. 2018 [cited 2019, Apr 9]. Essential Public Health Functions, Health Systems and Health Security: Developing Conceptual Clarity and a WHO Roadmap for Action [Internet]. Available from: https://apps.who.int/iris/handle/10665/272597
6. Appleyard J, Botbol M, Epperly T, Ghebrehiwet T, Grove J, Mezzich JE, Rawaf S, Salloum IS, Snaedal J, Van Dulmen S. 2016. Patterns and Prospects for the Implementation of Person-Centered Primary Care and People-Centered Public Health. International Journal of Person Centered Medicine 6 (1): 9–17.
7. Institute of Medicine (US) Committee for the Study of the Future of Public Health. 1988 [cited 2019, Apr 10]. The Disarray of Public Health: A Threat to

the Health of the Public [Internet]. Washington, DC: National Academies Press (US). Available from: https://www.ncbi.nlm.nih.gov/books/NBK218222

8. Morens DM, Fauci AS. 2013. Emerging Infectious Diseases: Threats to Human Health and Global Stability. PLOS Pathogens 9 (7): e1003467.

9. Cohen D, Huynh T, Sebold A, Harvey J, Neudorf C, Brown A. 2014 Feb 7 [cited 2019, Apr 22]. The Population Health Approach: A Qualitative Study of Conceptual and Operational Definitions for Leaders in Canadian Healthcare. SAGE Open Med [Internet] 2. Available from: https://www.ncbi.nlm.nih.gov/pmc/articles/PMC4607218

10. Health Canada. 2001 [cited 2019, Apr 1]. The Population Health Template: Key Elements and Actions That Define a Population Health Approach: July 2001 Draft [Internet]. Ottawa, ON. 42 p. Available from: http://www.phac-aspc.gc.ca/ph-sp/pdf/discussion-eng.pdf

11. Kindig D, Stoddart G. 2003. What Is Population Health? American Journal of Public Health 93 (3): 380–383.

12. Farmanova E, Baker GR, Cohen D. 2019. Combining Integration of Care and a Population Health Approach: A Scoping Review of Redesign Strategies and Interventions, and Their Impact. International Journal of Integrated Care [Internet] 19(2). Available from: https://www.ncbi.nlm.nih.gov/pmc/articles/PMC6460499

13. DeSalvo KB, Wang YC, Harris A, Auerbach J, Koo D, O'Carroll P. 2017 [cited 2019, May 6]. Public Health 3.0: A Call to Action for Public Health to Meet the Challenges of the 21st Century. Preventing Chronic Disease [Internet] 14. Available from: https://www.ncbi.nlm.nih.gov/pmc/articles/PMC5590510

14. Cloninger CR, Salvador-Carulla L, Kirmayer, LJ, Schwartz MA, Appleyard J, Goodwin N, Groves J, Hermans MHM, Mezzich JE, van Staden CW, Rawaf S. 2014. A Time for Action on Health Inequities: Foundations of the 2014 Geneva Declaration on Person- and People-Centered Integrated Health Care for All. International Journal of Person Centered Medicine 4: 69–89.

15. Mezzich JE, Kirisci L, Salloum I, Trivedi J, Kar SK, Adams N, Wallcraft J. 2016. Systematic Conceptualization of Person Centered Medicine and Development and Validation of a Person-Centered Care Index. International Journal of Person Centered Medicine 6: 219–247. Available from: http://www.ijpcm.org/index.php/IJPCM/article/view/219-247

16. Deau X, Appleyard J. 2015. Person Centered Medicine as an Ethical Imperative. International Journal of Person Centered Medicine 5(2): 60–63.

17. H. Barrett D, W. Ortmann L, Dawson A, Saenz C, Reis A, Bolan G, editors. 2016 [cited 2019, Sep 29]. Public Health Ethics: Cases Spanning the Globe [Internet]. Cham: Springer International Publishing. (Public Health Ethics

Analysis;   vol.   3).   Available   from: http://link.springer.com/10.1007/978-3-319-23847-0

18. Pan American Health Organization. 2012 [cited 2019, Jul 29]. Bioethics: Towards the Integration of Ethics in Health [Internet]. 28th Pan American Sanitary Conference, 64th Session of the Regional Committee of WHO for the Americas: Pan American Health Organization. Available from: http://iris.paho.org/xmlui/handle/123456789/49481

19. Rehfuess EA, Stratil JM, Scheel IB, Portela A, Norris SL, Baltussen R. 2019. The WHO-INTEGRATE Evidence to Decision Framework Version 1.0: Integrating WHO Norms and Values and a Complexity Perspective. BMJ Global Health 4 (Suppl 1): e000844.

20. Thomas JC, Sage M, Dillenberg J, Guillory VJ. 2002. A Code of Ethics for Public Health. American Journal of Public Health 92 (7): 1057–1059.

21. Institute of Medicine. 2012 [cited 2018, Oct 30]. Primary Care and Public Health: Exploring Integration to Improve Population Health [Internet]. Washington, DC: National Academies Press. Available from: https://www.nap.edu/catalog/13381/primary-care-and-public-health-exploring-integration-to-improve-population

22. White F. 2015. Primary Health Care and Public Health: Foundations of Universal Health Systems. Medical Principles and Practice 24 (2): 103–116.

23. Macinko JA, Montenegro Arriagada H, Nebot C, Pan American Health Organization. 2007. Renewing Primary Health Care in the Americas: A Position Paper of the Pan American Health Organization/World Health Organization (PAHO/WHO). Washington, DC: Pan American Health Organization.

24. Korc M, Hubbard S, Suzuki T, Jimba M. 2016 [cited 2019, Sep 24]. Health, Resilience, and Human Security: Moving toward Health for All. Japan Center for International Exchange, Pan American Health Organization. [Internet]. Available from: http://iris.paho.org/xmlui/handle/123456789/28286

SECTION 2

Communication, Common Ground, Diagnosis, and Assessment

EDITORIAL INTRODUCTION

ICPCM EDUCATIONAL PROGRAM ON PERSON-CENTERED CARE: COMMUNICATION, COMMON GROUND, DIAGNOSIS, AND ASSESSMENT

W. James Appleyard, MA, MD, FRCP[a] and
Juan E. Mezzich, MD, MA, MSc, PhD[b]

Keywords: person-centered Medicine, educational program, person-centered care, International College of Person Centered Medicine, communication, establishing common ground, collaborative assessment, clinical interviewing, person-centered diagnosis, continuity and integration of assessment and care, life cycle

Correspondence Address: Prof. W. James Appleyard, Thimble Hall Blean Common, Kent CT2 9JJ, United Kingdom

E-mail: jimappleyard2510@aol.com

INTRODUCTION

This volume includes the second set of papers that comprise the Educational Program on Person-Centered Care of the International College of Person Centered Medicine (ICPCM).

Person-centeredness is the foundation of the patient physician relationship, which is itself at the heart of medical practice and health care. This relationship is based on the dialogue between the patient as a person and the physician as a

---

[a] *Board Adviser and Former President, International College of Person Centered Medicine; Former President, World Medical Association; Former President, International Association of Medical Colleges*
[b] *Professor of Psychiatry, Icahn School of Medicine at Mount Sinai, New York; Hipólito Unanue Chair of Person Centered Medicine, San Marcos National University, Lima; Former President, World Psychiatric Association; Secretary General and Former President, International College of Person Centered Medicine*

professional person, allowing trust to develop between these two individuals so that the best interest of the person can be jointly sought through shared decision making within a clearly understood ethical framework. The Art of Medicine involves the application of knowledge and skills within this framework of collective conscience to make a judgment in the best interest of an individual seeking care. Communication is the life blood of this professional dialogue. Physicians and all health care professionals should always be able to cultivate empathy with a person seeking their help, respect the dignity of the individual, and demonstrate the ability to recognize and understand in the unfolding narrative the continuing interaction between psyche (mind, spirit) and soma (body).

COMMUNICATION

The theme of communication runs through each of the papers in this part of the Educational Program. Treating patients as persons, by considering their individual level of understanding, self-management skills, concerns, and care preferences, is central to our thinking. Yet, in medical practice, such an approach is not easy, as many other obligations and formalities intrude distracting attention from the person behind the patient. Many patients continue to experience barriers while communicating with their health care professionals [1]. For this reason, numerous interventions have been developed and implemented to optimize health care professionals' attitudes and communication skills to really engage with a patient, and to strengthen a patient's communication skills in order to be heard and understood.

For instance, in a detailed analysis of the interviews of patients four clinically relevant themes emerged – being treated as a person, being treated as an equal, being treated as the physician would want to be treated, and being cared about. Conducting a respectful physician–patient encounter does not necessarily involve complex interventions. Subtle, often nonverbal communicative behaviors, such as being polite, listening to the patient, being honest, and allowing a patient's input, can already turn a business-like patient encounter into a respectful, person-centered visit from which both the patient and the physician will benefit.

Medically unexplained physical symptoms (MUPS) [2] burden patients in their well-being and functioning and have a prevalence of approximately 25–50% in primary and specialist care. Physicians and other health care professionals often find patients with unexplained symptoms difficult to manage and the patients are not always understood. They are very well able to exclude diseases in case of symptoms that are not easily understood. Yet, they experience difficulties in explaining MUPS in terms of perpetuating factors and in motivating patients for therapy aimed at limiting the consequences of symptoms in case of moderate and persistent MUPS. Since there are various MUPS explanations and approaches, patients easily get confused by different and sometimes inconsistent messages from doctors and hence clear communication at the interface between primary and secondary care is necessary. Explaining MUPS in a person-centered way, answering GPs' referral questions and patients' questions, and giving a clear advice to patient and GP could improve MUPS specialist care and positively influence patient outcomes.

Physicians must engage in a true partnership with their patients as unique individuals always considering the social determinants of health specific to each person and context. Important attributes of the physician include listening and looking attentively with the ability to adapt and personalize each anamnesis and physical examination relevant to the individual person.

THE PERSON-CENTERED PHYSICIAN

Person-centered medicine involves physicians treating patients as whole human beings rather than as a symptom, collection of symptoms or a disease [3]. He or she needs to be approachable, interested, and inspire confidence, so that showing compassion and caring may absorb people's pain and anxieties without losing focus. It takes time to listen and communicate honestly and effectively with patients, relatives, staff teams, managers, peers, and local and national dignitaries pitched at the appropriate level while putting everyone at ease. Within a supporting clinical team, it is essential to show respect for all its members, and to know their names, their capabilities, and their contribution to the team, as well as to be fair and nonjudgmental.

The evidence for the application of a physician's knowledge and technical skills must be clear within the context of the individual patient. The physician needs to be able to synthesize conflicting and incomplete information, and to deal with uncertainty before reaching a probable diagnosis. Protocols and guidelines abound but physicians often must work outside these in the best interests of patients, as they express them; for example, when the best treatment for one condition may make a coexisting condition worse.

Physicians in their everyday practice have to manage risk. Many patients are alive today because doctors took risks. Physicians need to bring all their professional experience to bear on knowing when acceptable, informed, and carefully considered risk ends and recklessness begins – and share that information openly and honestly with their patients, always respecting that the final decision is the patient's, yet carrying and accepting ultimate responsibility for their professional actions.

Physicians need to recognize that change both in medicine and society is constant and ensure that professional standards, which are fundamental, are preserved while those practices that are simply a product of their time are allowed to lapse. They should have the ability to remain calm and proficient when under pressure and still make clear and timely decisions on behalf of their patients.

Physicians should be altruistic and visionary leaders who are competent and confident about their standards and steadfastly maintain their own and the team's professional values. They should be inspiring, always learning and teaching without fear of being proved wrong or being humiliated. They should show leadership and at the same time work collegially with all members of the health team.

THE RELEVANCE OF MEDICAL EDUCATION

In order to take positive action to implement a return to person-centered medicine, it is important to focus particularly on all stages of a physician's education including the selection of medical students. The selection of medical students has been conventionally done almost exclusively on the basis of measurements of knowledge and skills relevant to purely scientific disciplines. Indeed, a recently published statement on the core values and attributes needed to study medicine in the United Kingdom entitled "Selecting for Excellence" [4] itemizes 17 key skills and attributes – 16th in the list is "empathy and the ability to care for others" and at the bottom of the list is "honesty" – an attribute essential for a physician's integrity!

There needs to be a shift to a greater emphasis on the student's humanistic values and aptitude, recognizing the key importance of the ethical basis of the patient–physician relationship, the autonomy of the person seeking professional help, and each person's biological, psychosocial, and spiritual dimensions.

The WMA Statement on Medical Education and the Selection of Medical Students [5] states that following:

"A general liberal education is beneficial for anyone embarking on the study of medicine. A broad cultural education in the arts, humanities, and social sciences, as well as biological and physical sciences, is advantageous. Students should be chosen for the study of medicine on the basis of their intellectual ability, motivation, previous experiences, and character and integrity. The numbers admitted for training must meet the needs of the population and be matched by appropriate resources. Selection of students should not be influenced by age, sex, race, creed, political persuasion or national origin, although the mix of students should reflect the population."

The focus of student selection should shift to the student's humanistic values and aptitude, respect for the human rights of all people, attention to the important dynamic of a person's "flesh and spirit," its relation to families and professional environment, and the patient's autonomy and freedom of choice recognizing the centrality of the dialogue between the physician and the patient with shared decision making. The disciplines of sociology and philosophy should be given equal emphasis as the purely scientific disciplines. Learning from patients is an essential part of a physician's early and continuing education and the person-centered approach should be mandatory since the early professional years before proceeding to specializations.

The doctor–patient relationship demands the constant improvement of a physician's interpersonal skills, enabling the appropriate application of a physician's knowledge and skills. Person-centeredness based on the medical profession's ethical commitments must permeate all aspects of a physician's continuing education so that it becomes an internalized ethical duty for all practitioners of medicine.

THE QUALITY OF HEALTH CARE

Effective person-centered communication is the cornerstone of patient safety and the quality of health care. Poor physician–patient and health team communication is the underlying cause for nearly 66% of all medical errors [6]. This "patient as a person" communication diminishes the number and type of complaints and claims to physicians [7], producing in physicians greater well-being and less professional exhaustion. There is evidence that patients' perception of and satisfaction with the quality of the health care they experience depends on the quality of interactions with their health care professional. This relational approach also improves other clinical outcomes, referred to as diagnostic and therapeutic effectiveness – especially in chronic and cancer patients [8].

There is evidence of strong person-centered relationships between a health care team member's communication skills and a patient's capacity to adhere to medical recommendations, self-manage a chronic medical condition, and adopt preventive health behaviors. Effective person-centered care skills and attitudes among health care team members influence the quality of working relationships and job satisfaction [9]. When communication about tasks and responsibilities is done well, there is a significant reduction in nurse turnover and improved job satisfaction because it facilitates a culture of mutual support.

CLINICAL COMMUNICATION AND EMPATHY

In the first of the four papers included in this section of the monograph, Michel Botbol [10] emphasizes the relational and contextual elements of person-centered practice, the importance of empathy, attentiveness, and dialogue participation and empowerment. He asserts that clinical communication and empathy are essential in person-centered medicine being the conditions that recognize the patients' feelings, values, and expectations.

It is important to reflect on the processes allowing a professional to access these crucial dimensions through the development of a communication involving not only conscious or objective aspects, but also unconscious or subjective aspects. Empathy and narrative are the corner stone of this process.

The health professional should be trained to listen and attend to the verbal and nonverbal communication from patients and to build, in interaction with them, narratives giving access to their subjective dimensions.

COMMON GROUND FOR COLLABORATIVE CARE

The second paper Setting a Common Ground for Collaborative Care and Clinical Interviewing by Juan E. Mezzich [11] aims at articulating the place, features, and value of relationships and collaboration for organizing all clinical care, including clinical interviewing. He found from a literature review that the broadest and most compelling factor for organizing clinical care effectively in general, and concerning interviewing, assessment and diagnosis in particular, seems to be the setting up of a collaborative common ground among clinicians, patient, and family. Also, crucial concerning diagnosis is that this should be seen fundamentally as a process and not just a label or a formulation. Historical and anthropological research elucidates health care as part of social cooperation for the preservation and promotion of life. More recent research is also supportive of the positive perceptions of clinicians on procedures that are culturally informed and consider personal experience and values.

PERSON-CENTRED INTEGRATIVE DIAGNOSIS

The third paper entitled "Person-Centered Integrative Diagnosis: Concepts and Procedures" by Ihsan Salloum and Juan E. Mezzich [12] illustrates how the person-centered integrative diagnosis (PID) model facilitates the implementation of person-centered medicine. It reflects the importance of incorporating the patient's experience, culture, and values into the *core* of clinical diagnosis through a health experience formulation, along with more conventional diagnostic aspects such as health status and health risk and protective factors.

The design of a person-centered integrative diagnosis (PID) model was based on literature reviews and work meetings in London, Paris, Geneva, Preston, UK, and Uppsala, Sweden. The current PID model is composed of the following three broad levels: health status (from disorders and disability to well-being, all measured with standardized instruments), health contributors (risk factors and protective factors), and health experience and values. It includes categorical, dimensional, and narrative elements and involves the interactive engagement of clinicians, patients, and families and other care givers.

The PID model provides a holistic and culturally informed model that emphasizes patients and stakeholder engagement and shared decision making and places the person in context at the center of assessment and care. Illustratively, the PID has been adopted as the basis of the Latin American Guide for Psychiatric Diagnosis published by the Latin American Psychiatric Association for the use of health professionals in that world region.

CONTINUITY AND INTEGRATION OF PERSON-CENTERED ASSESSMENT

The fourth paper "Continuity and Integration of Person-Centered Assessment and Care across the Life Cycle" [13] by J Appleyard and M Botbol reflects the importance of placing the person in the wider context of his or her life's journey recognizing that health is a consequence of multiple determinants operating in interrelated genetic, biological, behavioral, social, and economic contexts that change as a person develops. The timing and sequence of such events and experiences influence the health and development of both individuals and populations. The influence of early adverse factors has a profound effect on later stages of life.

The health and well-being of a person are complex adaptive processes related to the consequences of genetic, biological, social, cultural, behavioral, and economic determinants throughout the life course. A life course perspective offers a more joined up approach with significant implications for long-term health gain. There is an emphasis on an integrated continuum of early intervention and education rather than of disconnected and unrelated stages. Each stage in the life of a person exerts influence on the next.

Disparities in health outcomes and in the psychosocial factors contributing to them are present early in life and are expressed and compounded during a person's lifetime. Risk factors are embedded in a person's biological makeup, manifested in disparities in a population's health, and maintained by social, cultural, and economic forces. They advocate a three-dimensional picture of a person who evolves laterally in the present, longitudinally from earlier life events and likely future projections, and vertically from the advances in the medical sciences.

REFERENCES

1. Van Dulmen S. 2016. Person Centered Communication in Healthcare: A Matter of Reaching Out. International Journal of Person Centered Medicine 6: 30–31.
2. Weiland A, Blankenstein AH, van Saase JL, van der Molen HT, Kosak D, Vernhout RM, Arends LR. 2016. Training Medical Specialists in Communication about Medically Unexplained Physical Symptoms: Patient Outcomes from a Randomized Controlled Trial. International Journal of Person Centered Medicine 6: 50–60.
3. Mezzich JE, Appleyard JW, Botbol M. 2017. Engagement and Empowerment in Person Centered Medicine. International Journal of Person Centered Medicine 7: 1–4.
4. Selecting for Excellence. The Final Report 2016 Medical Schools Council UK. www.medschools.ac.uk
5. WMA Statement on Medical Education 2017. www.wma.net
6. Institute for Health Communication 2011. https://healthcarecomm.org/about-us/impact-of-communication-in-healthcare
7. Levinson W, Roter DL, Mullooly JP, Dull VT, Frankel RM. 1997. Physician-Patient Communication. The Relationship with Malpractice Claims among Primary Care Physicians and Surgeons. Journal of the American Medical Association 277: 553–559.
8. Stewart M, Brown JB, Donner A, McWhinney IR, Oates J, Weston WW, Jordan J. 2000. The Impact of Patient-Centered Care on Outcomes. Journal of Family Practice 49: 796–804.
9. Ruiz-Moral R, Perula de Torres LA, Jaramillo-Martin I. 2007. The Effect of Patients' Met Expectations on Consultation Outcomes. A Study with Family Medicine Residents. Journal of General Internal Medicine 22: 86–91.
10. Botbol M, Van Dulmen S. This issue. Communication and Empathy within Person-Centered Medicine: A Developmental Point of View. International Journal of Person Centered Medicine 8(3): 17–27.
11. Mezzich JE. This issue. Setting a Common Ground for Collaborative Care and Clinical Interviewing. International Journal of Person Centered Medicine 8(3): 29–40.

12. Salloum IM, Mezzich JE. This issue. Person-Centered Integrative Diagnosis: Concepts and Procedures. International Journal of Person Centered Medicine 8(3): 41–49.
13. Appleyard J, Botbol M. This issue. Continuity and Integration of Person-Centered Assessment and Care across the Life Cycle. International Journal of Person Centered Medicine 8(3): 51–59.

COMMUNICATION AND EMPATHY WITHIN PERSON-CENTERED MEDICINE: A DEVELOPMENTAL POINT OF VIEW

Michel Botbol, MD, MSc[a] and Sandra Van Dulmen, PhD[b]

ABSTRACT

Communication between patients and health care providers (HCP) is at the heart of medicine and even more within its person-centered paradigm. Within a person-centered medicine (PCM) perspective, it is thus crucial, for both the HCP and the patient, to build on a relationship with the objective to establish a therapeutic alliance and share decision making related to the patient's health issues and to integrate the subjective aspects (and not only the objective aspects) of these health issues.

After showing that the effects of communication go beyond mere cognitive and affective sharing, particularly in highly emotional relations, this paper's objective is to understand more thoroughly what is transmitted in the patients/HCP relation and how some of the child and adolescent developmental psychiatry processes (i.e., early mother–baby interactions and transgenerational transmission of attachment) provide good models to understand this transmission.

Building on these models, the paper will discuss how and at which conditions, the HCP's narrative empathy plays a major role to access to the patient's subjectivity through the HCP's subjective experience.

It concludes that, therefore, subjectivity of the HCPs should not be seen as a negative side effect of the patient–HCP (or the patient–team) relation but as a crucial clinical tool in person-centered diagnostics and cares if HCPs are properly trained and educated to use their feelings and representations as tools in individual

[a] *Board of Directors, International College of Person Centered Medicine; Secretary for Scientific Publications, World Psychiatric Association; Emeritus Professor of Child and Adolescent Psychiatry, University of Western Brittany, Brest, France*
[b] *Professor, NIVEL (Netherlands Institute for Health Services Research), Utrecht, The Netherlands; Department of Primary and Community Care, Radboud University Medical Center, Nijmegen, The Netherlands; and Buskerud and Vestfold University College, Drammen, Norway*

or collective deliberations. But one has to be aware that there is no empathy without subjectivity.

Keywords: communication, empathy, person-centered medicine, attachment, subjectivity, narratives, metaphorizing empathy

Correspondence Address: Prof. Michel Botbol, 20 rue Littré, 75006 Paris, France

E-mail: botbolmichel@orange.fr

BACKGROUND

According to McCormack et al. [1], person-centeredness is "an approach to clinical practice that is established through the formation and fostering of therapeutic relationships underpinned by values of respect for persons and the individual right to self-determination, mutual respect and understanding." Recently, the term "therapeutic relationships" has been changed to "healthful relationships" [2], which are relationships that contribute to the promotion of health.

Communication between patients and health care providers (HCPs) is at the heart of medicine and even more so within this adapted person-centered paradigm. In person-centered medicine, the person of the patient comes first. This means that when someone seeks health care, his or her needs, preferences, beliefs, and values should also be considered when discussing complaints and considering a treatment. Person-centered communication allows the patient to express experiences, thoughts, and ideas, and makes it possible for the HCP to adapt the communication to the patient's emotional and informational needs [3].

Following person-centered principles, equal attention is given to the frequency and severity of physical symptoms as to persons' (and their carers') experiences and concerns evoked by these symptoms. Apart from that, positive health-related aspects, reflected for instance in a person's resilience, extended social network, positive mood, and healthy lifestyle, are taken in consideration as well.

When HCPs and patients meet, all these aspects need to be discussed as part of a "healthful relationship." Obviously, this places high demands on the communication skills and attitudes of the HCP. Being trained to solve medical problems HCP can experience feelings of uncertainty and of loss of control when they shift to a more egalitarian HCP-patient interaction in which treatment decision making and adherence depend much more on reaching consensus than on simply providing unidirectional advice. Yet, in person-centered medicine, the person of the HCP counts as much as that of the patient.

Daily confrontations with pain and suffering can make HCPs vulnerable, stressed, and sometimes even indifferent. Although such mechanisms are understandable and sometimes even self-protecting, they also appear to be associated with a higher risk of burn-out, job satisfaction, and suboptimal care [4]. Remarkably, the answer to the question on how to avoid these negative effects lies in the problem itself. Although it may be hard and counterproductive for HCPs to show compassion with patients in their everyday work, it can also protect them from becoming too stressed and indifferent. Research shows that being compassionate and involved in meaningful relationships with patients may even contribute to the well-being of a HCP [5]. Being compassionate and involved is not the only way to go. Self-compassion, and self-understanding also seems to be associated with HCPs experiencing more positive work engagement, feeling less emotionally, physically, and cognitively exhausted due to work demands, and being more satisfied with work [6]. This indicates the importance of not only taking care of one's patients and of maintaining a good HCP–patient relationship but also of taking good care of oneself as HCP. This underlines the importance of looking after both persons involved in a health care relation: the person of the patient and the person of the HCP.

Within a person-centered medicine (PCM) perspective, it is thus crucial for both the HCP and the patient to build on a relationship with the objective (1) to establish a therapeutic alliance and share decision making related to the patient's health issues and (2) to integrate the subjective aspects (and not only the objective aspects) of these health issues.

This paper will discuss how and at which conditions, communication and empathy play a crucial role to reach this objective.

COMMUNICATION

In a narrow sense, communication has been defined as the transmission of cognitive information through language (mainly verbal). More broadly defined, it also includes [7]:

- Digital and analogic (verbal and nonverbal) transmission
- Emotional and cognitive dimensions
- Contextualized and interactive relations

There is ample evidence for the importance of this broad definition in clinical situations, e.g., the length of time a patient is listened to before being interrupted by the professional, changes drastically the patient's experience of the medical interview (i.e., his feeling of being understood by the professional increases when the longer he is allowed to talk) [8–10].

Additionally, many researchers consider that the effects of communication go beyond mere cognitive and affective sharing, particularly in highly emotional relations, that is to say in relations involving the intense feeling of understanding and sharing with the other [7].

Patient–professional (or carers) relations are frequently highly emotional, allowing them to include a holistic appraisal of the person of the patient through the creation of a more or less temporary common space. In this common space the border between the patient and the professional (or carers) is temporarily porous and confused. However, they are not eradicated, i.e., they do not lose sight of the otherness of the other (its "alterity"). Yet, communication does not take place in a vacuum but is part of a context [11].

MODELS OF TRANSMISSION

To understand more thoroughly what is – besides the communication of cognitive and affective information – transmitted, other less well-known theoretical models can be helpful. Child and adolescent developmental psychiatry provides such models among which two are particularly relevant:

- The model of early mother–baby interactions in the subjectivation process
- The model of the transgenerational transmission of attachment

1. The model of early mother–baby interactions in the subjectivation process

This model aims to explain how babies evolve from a fusional state to individuation and subjectivation, and how this process develops in the "mother"–baby interactions at an early stage of the baby's life (fig.1) [12]. It also helps to explain how, in this process, babies acquire very complex and sophisticated social abilities on the basis of rather simple and limited innate abilities. It is an example of the type of process Berthoz named "Simplexity" [13].

Three dimensions are involved in these interactions (12): (1) behavioral: the body, the voice, the gaze; (2) affective: progressive affective attunement; and (3) imaginary (fig. 2).

The interactions pertaining to the imaginary dimensions are not objective but, nevertheless, conceptually necessary to describe what is happening in the mother–baby or the parent–baby dyad: an interaction of conscious and unconscious representations. The interactions pertaining to these dimensions give also access to transgenerational and cultural influences through the parents, whatever are the biological mechanisms supporting this transmission.

The addition of this third dimension introduces a crucial conceptual complexification of the subjectivation process and can explain how a rather simple

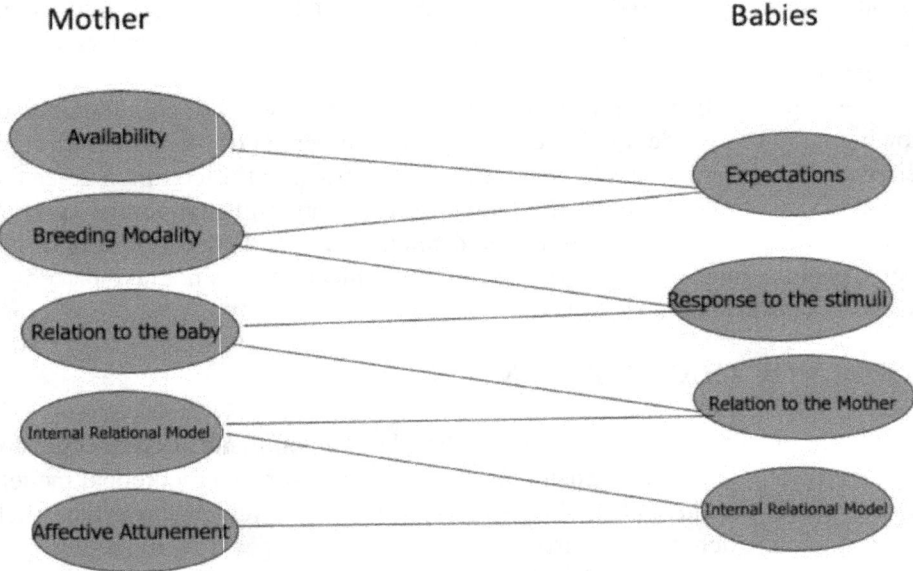

Figure 1. Early interactions: the Bobigny Model (Lebovici)

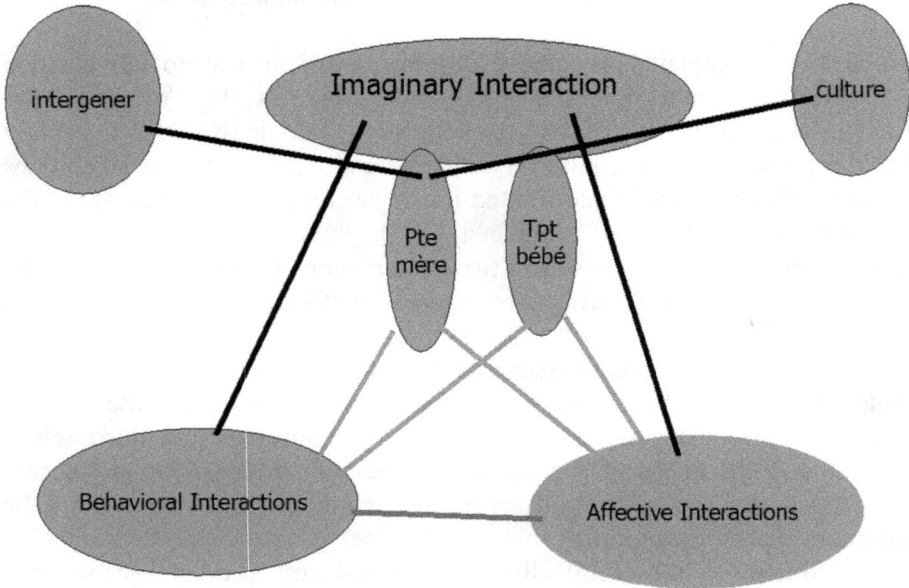

Figure 2. The three dimensions involved in early interactions

process (as everyday behavioral and affective interactions) can lead to the transmission of very sophisticated and complex dimensions and values, on the ground of baby's innate intersubjective capacities [14].

With the addition of the imaginary dimensions to the behavioral and affective interactions, communication undergoes a qualitative conceptual leap making it complex enough to transmit sophisticated subjective dimensions and values, through basic interactions.

2. The model of the transgenerational transmission of attachment

Attachment is a psychological notion aiming to describe the dynamic of interpersonal relationship on the basis of a behavioral and mental system directing the infant to seek proximity with the main attachment figure, generally one of the parents, whenever in a separation or alarming situation. Bowlby who was a well-known British psychoanalyst built a developmental theory on this notion [15], extending to the human infant what has been observed by ethologist in primates: a primary attachment system developing in the first year of the infant life on the basis of common innate needs expressed and taking various forms according to the style of attachment; this style results from the autoregulation provided by a set of mental representation Bowlby calls Internal Working Models.

Protocols and instruments were created by Bowlby's followers to evaluate these styles (i.e., The Strange Situation Protocol – SSP – in infants, and the Adult Attachment Interview – AAI – in Adults). These standardized instruments defined four dimensions of attachment [16]:

* Secure (AAI and SSP)
* Detached (AAI) or Avoidant (SSP)
* Preoccupied (AAI) or Ambivalent (SSP)
* Disorganized (AAI and SSP)

Additionally, further studies showed a strong correlation between the pattern of attachment of the mother (evaluated by the AAI) and the pattern of attachment of her infant (evaluated by the SSP). The finding that this strong correlation was not related to genetic transmission nor to the mere sensitivity of the attachment figures generated numerous theories and studies around what was then known as the "transmission gap." This soon became one of the main paradigms for examining the nongenetic transgenerational transmission in parents–infant's early relations [16].

Tackling this important issue, several studies brought converging clues on the role of microbehaviors in the transgenerational transmission [17]: while engaged in the highly emotional relation an infant has with his mother, he is sensitive to the microbehavior he observes on his mother's' face; to the point that he simulates them (using probably his mirror neurons system) [18]. This simulation acts as a template on which he will build up his capacity to recognize emotions and their meaning, constructing his Internal Working Model on his "lived experience of invariably repeated schemes of interactions with the attachment object" [19]. In this perspective, the infant behavioral pattern of attachment would be the basis on which the Internal Working Model is built rather than the contrary. This model generates clear hypotheses to examine and embody, at a fine-grained level, the mechanisms of the transmission of attachment. Mutatis mutandis, it can also be a good candidate to shed light on the mechanisms involved in the interaction between two persons engaged in a highly emotional relation, reminding us of the frequently quoted statement by Shore [20]: "The child's first relationship, the one with the mother, acts as a template that permanently molds the individual's capacity to enter into all later emotional relationships. Small children look to a parent's facial expressions and other nonverbal signals to determine how to respond and feel in a strange or ambiguous situation; it is the basis of empathy," in other words, a basis for social neuroscience.

PRACTICAL APPLICATION FOR PERSON-CENTERED MEDICINE

As mentioned above, integrating personal subjectivity is a categorical objective of person-centered medicine (PCM). In this perspective, subjectivity is indeed a crucial part of the patient's assessment and of the HCP's engagement in his cares. However, subjectivity is not easy to measure or assess objectively and is therefore frequently neglected or even rejected by evidence-based medicine. It is one of the reasons why EBM tends to favor a disorder-centered perspective on health care.

One of the main endeavors of PCM is to address this issue, trying to find a "scientific" or at least "a nonmetaphysic" way to assess this hidden dimension in the patient, his carers, and the HCP. A starting point here is to describe as precisely as possible, how we do it naturally in settings in which – like in clinical situations – highly emotional relationships develop with highly complex ambivalent and regressive components of dependency (fig.3) [21].

FIRST STEP: EMOTIONAL EMPATHY

Defined as the feelings induced by the contact with the patient through verbal and behavioral interactions, it is favored by "the affective permeability" induced by the process of constructing a common space in highly emotional contexts. We see it as the first methodological step to go behind the screen of the visible and a holistic way to approach subjectivity of the other as a holistic dimension.

SECOND STEP: METAPHORIZATION AND NARRATIVES

When the emotions behind the feelings are not actively rejected, the HCP captures these in narratives through his capacity to metaphorize these emotions and affects (put them into a story). These stories are of crucial importance because they are the best way for the HCP to access, acknowledge, and give meaning to his empathic subjective feelings. These narratives integrate (but are not reduced to) the patient's narratives to which the professional has to be attentive enough to include them among the data he "naturally" considers in the construction of his narrative.

This second step can then be defined as the transformation of Emotional Mirror Empathy into a Narrative (or Metaphorizing) Empathy [12]; it uses the professionals' representations and affects to approach and understand the patient subjectivity and integrate it in the assessment of his health status and shared decision making concerning his treatment.

THIRD STEP: WORKING THROUGH

To develop his narratives, the professional uses his idiosyncratic sensitivity to

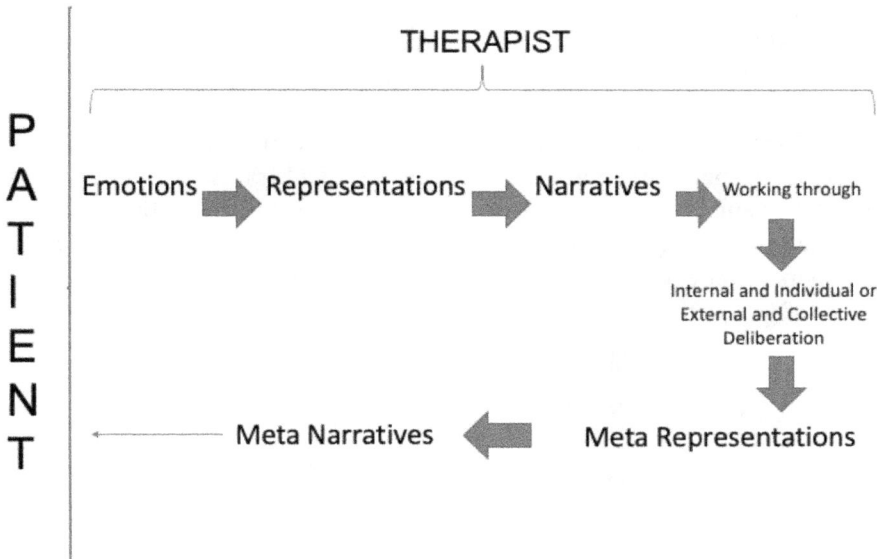

Figure 3. Narrative empathy process

recognize and highlight specific aspects of the patient's subjective life. It is acceptable as long as the professional keeps in mind that this story is a construction, which he has to control and work through in his internal deliberation. The same is true, also, in an institutional setting where each team member uses his idiosyncratic sensitivity to enrich specific aspects of the patient's subjective life, leading to a collective deliberation through the team work. In both situations, the final product of this individual or collective deliberations is the development of a meta-narrative integrating more or less of each of the contribution to the development of the current state of the narrative on and with the patient.

It is the closest we can get to the double constraints we have to face to integrate subjectivity in a PCM perspective:

- Reduction of the ill-effect of eradicating the patient's subjective idiosyncratic feelings, particularly those remaining unexpressed or unconscious;
- Reduction of the ill-effect of idiosyncratic sensitivity of the professionals when they are abusively considered as a final truth.

CONCLUSIONS

Subjectivity of the HCPs is not only a negative side effect of the patient–HCP (or the patient–team) relation; it is also a crucial clinical tool in person-centered diagnostics and cares and should therefore be analyzed and controlled, with HCPs properly trained to use their feelings and representations as tools in individual or collective deliberations. Empathy is a crucial tool here: but we have to be aware that there is no empathy without subjectivity; in PCM, subjectivity of the HCP is crucial too. This has crucial consequences for clinical practices and organizations, particularly regarding medical and HCPs' education and training; instead of the tendency of current classical curricula to ignore the subjective dimensions in medicine at large – leaving the HCPs and carers alone to deal with it, in themselves and in the person they are attending –, medical education should recognize the importance of subjectivity in a person-centered perspective, and integrate a training to use and regulate properly the subjectivity of the HCPs.

ACKNOWLEDGMENTS AND DISCLOSURES

The author does not report any conflicts of interest.

REFERENCES

1. McCormack B, Dewing J, McCance T. 2011. Developing Person-Centred Care: Addressing Contextual Challenges through Practice Development. Online Journal of Issues in Nursing 16 (2): 3.
2. McCormack B, McCance T. 2016. Person-Centred Practice in Nursing and Health Care: Theory and Practice, (2nd ed), Wiley Blackwell, Oxford.
3. Eide H, Eide T. 2007. Kommunikasjon i relasjoner. Samhandling, konfliktløsning, etikk [Communication in Relationships], (2nd ed), Gyldendal Academic Press, Oslo.
4. Bensing JM, van den Brink-Muinen A, Boerma W, van Dulmen S. 2013. The Manifestation of Job Satisfaction in Doctor-Patient Communication: A Ten-Country European Study. International Journal of Person Centered Medicine 3: 44–52.
5. Smith-MacDonald L, Venturato L, Hunter P, Kaasalainen S, Sussman T, McCleary L, Thompson G, Wickson-Griffiths A, Sinclair S. 2019. Perspectives and Experiences of Compassion in Long-Term Care Facilities within Canada: A Qualitative Study of Patients, Family Members and Health Care Providers. BMC Geriatrics 19 (1): 128.
6. Babenko O, Mosewich AD, Lee A, Koppula S. 2019. Association of Physicians' Self-Compassion with Work Engagement, Exhaustion, and Professional Life Satisfaction. Medical Sciences (Basel) 7 (2): 29.
7. Cosnier J. 2014. Communication et empathie [Communication and Empathy]. In: M Botbol, N Garret, & A Besse (Eds). L'Empathie au Carrefour de la Science et de la Clinique [Empathy at the Crossroad of Science and Clinics], Doin, Paris.
8. Marvel MK, Epstein RM, Flowers K, Beckman HB. 1999. Soliciting the Patient's Agenda. Have We Improved? Journal of the American Medical Association 281: 283–287.
9. Van Dulmen AM, Bensing JM. 2002. Health Promoting Effects of the Physician-Patient Encounter. Psychology, Health & Medicine 7: 289–300.
10. Langewitz W, Denz M, Keller A, Kiss A, Rüttimann S, Wössmer B. 2002. Spontaneous Talking Time at Start of Consultation in Outpatient Clinic: Cohort Study. British Medical Journal 28: 682–683.
11. Bensing JM, Dulmen AM van, Tates K. 2003. Communication in Context: New Directions in Communication Research. Patient Education and Counseling 50: 27–32.
12. Lebovici S. 1999. Arbre de vie: Éléments de Psychopathologie du Bébé bébé [The Tree of Life: Principles of Infant Psychopathology], Eres, Toulouse.
13. Berthoz A. 2009. La Simplexité. Odile Jacob, Paris.

14. Emde RN. 2016. From a Baby Smiling: Reflections on Virtues in Development. In: J Annas, D Narvaez, & NE Snow (Eds). Developing the Virtues: Integrating Perspectives. Oxford University Press, Oxford, pp. 69–94.

15. Bowlby J. 1999 [1969]. Attachment. Attachment and Loss (vol. 1). (2nd ed.), Basic Books, New York.

16. Fonagy P, Target M. 2005. Bridging the Transmission Gap: An End to an Important Mystery of Attachment Research? Attachment & Human Development 7: 333–343.

17. Botbol M. 2010. Towards an Integrative Neuroscientific and Psychodynamic Approach to the Transmission of Attachment. Journal of Physiology-Paris 104 (5): 263–271.

18. Iacoboni M. 2009. The Problem of Other Minds Is Not a Problem: Mirror Neurons and Intersubjectivity. In: J Pineda (Ed). Mirror Neuron Systems, Humana Press, New York, pp. 121–134.

19. Fonagy P. 2001. Développement de la Psychopathologie de l'Enfance à l'Age Adulte: Le mystérieux déploiement des Troubles dans le temps. La psychiatrie de l'enfant, 2 (44): 333–369.

20. Shore R. 1997. What Have We Learned? In: Rethinking the Brain, Families and Work Institute, New York, pp. 15–27.

21. Botbol M, Lecic Tosevski D. 2013. Person Centered Medicine and Subjectivity. In: JHD Cornelius-White, et al. (Eds), Interdisciplinary Applications of the Person-Centered Approach, Springer Science+Business Media, New York.

SETTING A COMMON GROUND FOR COLLABORATIVE CARE AND CLINICAL INTERVIEWING

Juan E. Mezzich, MD, MA, MSc, PhD[a]

ABSTRACT

Background: A relationship and communication matrix and collaborative assessment and care, as part of a set of elicited principles and strategies, are hallmarks of person-centered medicine and health care. Their formulation and cultivation have been predicated on both humanistic and scientific grounds.
Objectives: This paper is aimed at articulating the bases, key concepts, and strategies for establishing common ground among clinicians, patient, and family for organizing all person-centered clinical care, starting with clinical interviews.
Method: For addressing these objectives, a selective review of the clinical literature was conducted. This was complemented by contrasting the findings with the results of similar papers and reflecting on their implications.
Results: One of the broadest and most compelling factors for organizing person-centered clinical care effectively in general, and particularly concerning interviewing, assessment, and diagnosis as well as treatment planning and implementation, seems to be setting up *common ground* among clinicians, patient, and family. Crucial dynamic matrices of common ground seem to be (1) assembling and engaging the key players for effective care, (2) establishing empathetic communication among these players, (3) organizing participative diagnostic processes toward joint understanding of the presenting person's personhood and health (both problems and positive aspects), and (4) planning and implementing clinical care through shared decision making and joint commitments. Critical guiding considerations for common ground appear to include holistic informational integration, taking into consideration the person's chronological and space context, and attending to his or her health experience, preferences, and values. Among the

[a] *Professor of Psychiatry, Icahn School of Medicine at Mount Sinai, New York; Hipolito Unanue Professor of Person Centered Medicine, San Fernando Faculty of Medicine, San Marcos National University, Lima; Secretary General and Former President, International College of Person Centered Medicine; Former President, World Psychiatric Association*

most promising strategies for operationalizing common ground is the formulation of a narrative integrative synthesis of clinical and personal information as joint distillation of the assessment process and as foundation for planning care. These considerations also serve as framework for the delineation and organization of effective clinical interviewing.

Discussion: These findings are supported, first, by historical and anthropological research, which elucidates health care as part of social cooperation for the preservation and promotion of life. *Common ground* appears substantiated by the principles of person centered medicine, and represents one of its most clear projections. Also supportive of common ground is recent research on the positive perceptions of clinicians on procedures that are culturally informed and consider personal experience and values.

Conclusions: It appears that the establishment of a common ground among clinicians, patient, and family is a critical step for the effective person-centered organization of clinical care in general and for interviewing, diagnosis, and treatment planning in particular.

Keywords: common ground, collaborative care, clinical interviewing, assessment, comprehensive diagnosis, joint understanding, shared decision making, person-centered medicine

Conflicts of interest: The author reports no conflicts of interest.

Correspondence Address: Prof. Juan E. Mezzich, Icahn School of Medicine at Mount Sinai, Fifth Ave & 100 St., Box 1093, New York, New York 10029, USA

E-mail: juanmezzich@aol.com

BACKGROUND

While the simplest concept of person-centered medicine may involve putting *persons* first in health care, more considerate notions speak of having the person at the center of health [1, 2] and as the proper target of health actions [3]. Here the person is to be understood in a contextualized manner, as illustrated by Ortega y Gasset [4] aphorism "I am I and my circumstance; and if do not save it, I do not save myself." Furthermore, in specific reference to major aspects of the health field, conceptual outlines have been discussed over the years concerning person-centered clinical care [5] and people-centered public health [6].

Recent systematic explorations of person- and people-centered care through literature reviews and international consultations conducted by the International

College of Person Centered Medicine [7] have identified the following as key concepts: 1. Ethical commitment, 2. Holistic framework to understand health and illness, 3. Cultural awareness and responsiveness, 4. Communicational and relationship focus at all levels, 5. Individualization of care, 6. Establishment of common ground among clinicians, patient and family for collaborative diagnosis and shared decision making, 7. People-centered organization of integrated services, and 8. Person-centered health education and research.

Adams and Grieder [8], recognized experts on treatment planning, have posited *common ground* as the keystone for making such planning person-centered. Thus, to large degree, the above notions and principles of person-centered medicine would be relevant and helpful to understand the bases of establishing a common ground, substantiate its practical importance, and delineate its components and principal features.

OBJECTIVES

This paper is aimed at articulating the bases, features, and strategies for establishing a common ground among clinicians, patient, and family for organizing all clinical care in a person-centered manner, starting with clinical interviews.

METHOD

For addressing these objectives, a selective review of the clinical literature was conducted. This included particularly papers related to person-centered medicine and more generally literature involving clinical care with focus on relationship issues, communication, and collaborative care. This led to the identification of two sources specifically on common ground, two papers on communication and empathy germane to engagement for establishing common ground, two sources on person-centered diagnosis involving joint understanding of the clinical situation, and two sources on treatment planning involving shared decision making, which has common ground at its base. This was complemented with a comparison between the findings made and relevant perspectives in similar papers and reflecting on their implications. The reviewed papers are identified in the Results and the Discussion sections connected to the presented findings and reflections.

RESULTS

It has been proposed and demonstrated that the organization of person-centered clinical care should be substantiated and guided by philosophical and conceptual principles, giving attention to the personhood of the patients, health professionals,

83

and family members involved in caring for life and health [1]. Based on extensive clinical experience, Tempier [2] has proposed that "what is good for the persons is what is good for their health and mental health."

Among the key principles of person-centered medicine helpful to guide clinical care are those elucidated through systematic studies [7], which start with ethical commitment [9, 10]. This is usually formulated based on Aristotelian and Kantian insights as well as on fundamental human rights. The remaining principles are principally strategic and science-based.

One of them involves establishing common ground among health professionals, the patient and family members, in order to organize key clinical tasks in a collaborative fashion. These involve, first, the basic task of diagnosis aimed to the joint understanding of the clinical situation and not only the identification of existing illnesses, and second, collaborative treatment planning conducted as share decision making. The cruciality of establishing a common ground for person-centered care has been highlighted most cogently by Adams and Grieder [8].

Common Ground Matrices

The overarching strategy for establishing a common ground may be unpacked into a set of dynamic matrices as follows:

1. *Assembling and engaging the key players for effective care*

The individuals who tend to play a critical role in clinical care are the various involved clinicians representing different disciplines and specialties, the patient as the person presenting for evaluation and care, and the relevant family members. Specific players need to be pointedly identified and then engaged.

Concerning the collaborative clinician–patient relationship, Tasman [11] has cogently pointed out that this relationship must start since the first encounter and represents the fundamental matrix for the whole of care. The value of clinicians of various disciplines and specialties involved with a given patient to work coordinately with each other has been analyzed by Ghebrehiwet [12], who has pointed out that a well-articulated team approach is a hallmark of person-centered care. The need to foster communication among clinicians, patients, and families has been studied and advocated for by Amering [13].

2. *Establishing empathetic communication among key players*

The need to establish empathy in clinical communication appears to lead to a closer examination of the role of the professional's empathy in the methodology to access the subjectivity of the patient, as pointed out by Botbol and Lecic-Tosevski [14]. At first seen as the professional's ability to listen sympathetically to the comments of the patient and to consider his wishes and needs, the notion of empathy has gradually widened to include representations that the physician (or other health professional) makes of the clinical situation in which the person in need of care is involved. In short, these are representations that the professional makes of the health situation of the person suffering through the health professional's own empathy, triggered by the words and the acts of the patients and of their carers.

This mechanism is well described by the concept of "metaphorizing-empathy" proposed by Lebovici [15] from his work with babies and their mothers. It is also close to the notion of "narrative empathy" proposed by Hochmann [16] based on his work with autistic children and on the philosophical ideas brought up by Ricoeur [17] in his book "Time and Narrative." It is also consistent with Kleinman's [18] assumptions on illness narratives. This important development in person-centered medicine marks the full recognition of the role of the clinician's subjectivity as a diagnostic and treatment tool within the framework of the clinician–patient relationship.

3. *Organizing participative diagnostic processes*

The World Psychiatric Association (WPA) published in 2003 the International Guidelines for Diagnostic Assessment (IGDA) at the core of which is a diagnostic model articulating standardized multiaxial and idiographic personalized components [19]. These guidelines propose the interaction among clinicians, the patient, and the family to formulate together a joint statement on contextualized clinical problems, the patient's positive health, and expectations on health restoration and promotion. This diagnostic model has been applied in different countries as illustrated by the Latin American Guide for Psychiatric Diagnosis [20] and has been one of the starting points for the design of a Person-Centered Integrative Diagnosis model [21].

Addressing the nature of diagnosis, the eminent historian and philosopher of medicine Laín-Entralgo [22] cogently argued that diagnosis goes beyond identifying a disease (nosological diagnosis) to also involve understanding of what is going on in the body and mind of the person who presents for care. Diagnostic understanding also requires a process of engagement and empowerment that recognizes the agency of patient, family, and health professionals participating in a trialogical partnership [13].

4. *Planning and implementing clinical care through shared decision making and joint commitments*

Experienced clinicians suggest that treatment planning is the most important purpose of diagnosis [8]. In previous decades, the main purpose of diagnosis seemed to have been to identify an existing disorder and this informed the concept of validity of a diagnostic system. More recently, such validity concept, labeled "physio-pathogenic validity" is contrasted with an emerging one termed "clinical validity" related to value to inform clinical care [23]. The current edition of the American Psychiatric Association's [24] Diagnostic and Statistical Manual of Mental Disorders, DSM-5, is presented as principally aimed to assist clinical care. Furthermore, a survey among the members of the 43-country Global Network of National Classification and Diagnosis Groups [25] identified treatment planning as the key role of diagnosis.

It has been cogently argued that person-centered treatment and care must be made collaboratively among clinicians involved, the patient and his or her family. This collaborative approach is established for both diagnostic formulation and treatment planning by the Person-Centered Integrative Diagnosis model [21] and its practical application for Latin America, the GLADP-VR [26].

As pointed out by Adams [27], treatment plans are at the heart of any care process and are critical in guiding treatment decisions, as well as having an important role in patient engagement and treatment success. Adding to this, Arora and McHorney [28] have advised that treatment plans should be built upon and reflect both shared understanding and decision making between the patient and the health professional. Furthermore, shared understanding and shared decision making are to be rounded-up by the joint-commitment of all key players to the implementation and follow-up of treatment plans. Thus, all these crucial clinical care activities are to be built on common ground established among clinicians, patient, and family.

Guiding Considerations for Common Ground

Helpful guiding considerations for establishing *common ground,* adjusted from those outlined by Adams [27], may include the following:

1. *Holistic informational integration.* This is to be applied to the understanding of both illness and positive heath. It corresponds to one of the key principles of person-centered medicine as elucidated by Mezzich et al. [7].
2. *Addressing the person's longitudinal and cross-sectional context.* A contextualized concept of the whole person is at the core of person-centered medicine. It is predicated on the previously mentioned Ortega y Gasset's [4] dictum on circumstances that round-up the person's identity. Complementing this dictum, the scope of these circumstances may be optimized by referring

to both cross-sectional and longitudinal dimensions. The later extend from the person's historical roots and filiation to his or her life project [29].
3. *Attending to health experience, preferences, and values.* This feature brings to the front the key principles of person-centered medicine involving ethical commitment to the person's values [30] as well as that on cultural awareness and responsiveness [31, 32].

Common Ground Implementation

The operationalization or effective implementation of *common ground* may start with its first two dynamic matrices as outlined above, namely, (1) assembling and engaging the key players for effective care, and (2) establishing empathetic communication among them. The considerations formulated there are quite relevant as basic steps for common ground implementation. From the next two matrices of common ground, i.e., organizing participative diagnostic processes and cultivating shared decision making and joint commitments, emerge a promising collaborative activity and formulation, a *narrative integrative synthesis* of clinical and personal information as joint distillation of person-centered assessment processes and foundation of person-centered care planning.

One such synthesis was proposed as part of the International Guidelines for Diagnostic Assessment (IGDA) [19]. The comprehensive diagnostic statement included in the IGDA Guidelines encompassed a standard multiaxial formulation and, of particular relevance to common ground, a *personalized idiographic formulation.* The latter integrates the perspectives of the clinician, the patient, and the family into a jointly understood narrative summary of the clinical problems, the patient's positive points, and expectations for the restoration and promotion of health. It was presented as likely to be the most effective way to address the complexity of illness, the patient's whole health status and expectations, and their cultural framework.

Building on the above as well as on the more recent Person-Centered Integrative Diagnostic Model [21] and on a web approach to recovery and shared decision making [33], Adams [27] has articulated and illustrated with a detailed clinical case the essentials of an integrated narrative synthesis of the patient's clinical and personal data from a comprehensive diagnostic statement. Such a synthesis serves as a bridge between assessment and creation of a treatment plan and focuses on the value of a written narrative that captures the essence of joint understanding and the importance of dialog between key players that is the foundation of common ground.

Adams [27] points out that disagreement must be acknowledged and reconciled in the process, without which healing relationships may dissolve. The process of moving from mere information and ritualistic procedures to shared understanding, shared planning, and joint commitment is at the heart of what it means to be person-centered. Effective clinical solutions that are endorsed and supported by the patient may only come from this process.

Addressing the feasibility of such proposals, Adams indicates that bridging the gap between current conventional practice and what should be regular person-centered care practice is possible. Citing Davidson et al. [34], he submits that given adequate time for completing the integrative summary, along with the support and training necessary to include a formulation or narrative in the process of moving from assessment to creating treatment plans, many clinicians can develop the skills necessary to be more holistic and person-centered in routine care.

Toward a Person-Centered Clinical Interview

The considerations on common ground presented above may be helpful for setting the bases, organizing and conducting a person-centered clinical interview. The International Guidelines for Diagnostic Assessment (IGDA) [19] offer helpful guidelines.

The interview process should include a preparatory phase to ensure a quiet and reasonably comfortable environment where patients and families are received cordially and respectfully.

The body of the interview should cover in an effective, smooth, and considered manner the different areas of information relevant to an adequate diagnostic formulation and an initial treatment plan. It is essential to establish empathy, to attend to subjectivity and intersubjectivity, and to listen carefully to the patient and available family. This phase should conclude with the formulation of a jointly understood initial diagnostic assessment (which would continue later as the clinical care process unfolds), and shared decisions on what the next steps would be, as well as ensuring that the patient and family are aware, involved, and satisfied with such formulation.

The closure phase of the interview should include a warm farewell connected to future visits or clinical activities. It is important to conduct the interview in a respectful, warm, empathetic, and empowering manner.

DISCUSSION

The concepts and procedures presented in the preceding section appear to be consistent with or supported by the following perspectives and findings.

Historical and anthropological research, going back as much as that of Neanderthals, has described health care as integral part of social, small group, and family cooperation that were crucial for the preservation and promotion of life [35].

Common ground as a powerful factor for person-centered care appears substantiated by several principles of person-centered medicine (such as ethical commitment, holistic framework, cultural awareness and responsiveness, relationships and communication matrix, and collaborative care), and represents one of its most crucial applications and facilitators [9, 36, 37].

Also supportive of common ground is recent research on the positive perceptions of health professionals on clinical procedures that are culturally informed and consider personal experience and values [38].

CONCLUSIONS

Establishing *common ground* among health professionals, patient, and family for collaborative care appears to be at the core of the person-centered approach. It is consistent with most of the key principles of person-centered medicine and may be one of the most powerful factors to achieve person-centered care. Important and helpful information has been elucidated on the dynamic matrices where common ground plays, such as assembling key players for clinical care, promoting engagement and empathy among them, organizing participative comprehensive diagnosis, and shared decision making and commitment for health actions. Guiding considerations for establishing common ground have also been identified. Powerful strategies for implementing common ground have been outlined, particularly the collaborative formulation of an integrated narrative synthesis of the patient's clinical and personal information to serve as a bridge between assessment and the creation of a treatment plan. Within this general framework, an outline for the organization and conduction of clinical interviews has emerged.

ACKNOWLEDGMENTS AND DISCLOSURES

The author recognizes the important work of colleagues at the International College of Person Centered Medicine among many others. Their published contributions are formally referred to in the paper.

No conflicts of interest are reported.

REFERENCES

1. Cassell E. 2010. The Person in Medicine. International Journal of Integrated Care 10 (Suppl): 50–51.
2. Tempier R. 2010, September 1–5. Treatment and Care of Psychosis: The Person

First. Paper presented at Symposium on Person Centered Care, WPA Regional Meeting, Beijing.

3. Mezzich JE, Snaedal J, van Weel C, Heath I. 2010. Toward Person-Centered Medicine: From Disease to Patient to Person. Mount Sinai Journal of Medicine 77: 304–306.

4. Ortega y Gasset J. 1914. Meditaciones del Quijote. In: Obras Completas de José Ortega y Gasset. Madrid: Editorial Santillana, 2004, Vol 1, pp. 745–825.

5. Miles A, Mezzich JE. 2011. The Care of the Patient and the Soul of the Clinic: Person-Centered Medicine as an Emergent Model of Modern Clinical Practice. International Journal of Person Centered Medicine 1: 207–222.

6. WHO. 2009. Resolution of the General Assembly, WHO, Geneva.

7. Mezzich JE, Kirisci L, Salloum IM, Trivedi JK, Kar SK, Adams N, Wallcraft J. 2016. Systematic Conceptualization of Person Centered Medicine and Development and Validation of a Person-Centered Care Index. International Journal of Person Centered Medicine 6: 219–247.

8. Adams N, Grieder DM. 2005. Treatment Planning for Person-Centered Care, Elsevier, Amsterdam.

9. Appleyard J. 2013. Introduction to Ethical Standards for Person-Centered Health Research. International Journal of Person Centered Medicine 3: 258–262.

10. Bouësseau M-C. 2013. Strengthening Research Ethics Review Systems. International Journal of Person Centered Medicine 3: 263–265.

11. Tasman A. 2000. Presidential Address: The Doctor-Patient Relationship. American Journal of Psychiatry 157: 1763–1768.

12. Ghebrehiwet T. 2013. Effectiveness of Team Approach in Health Care: Some Research Evidence. International Journal of Person Centered Medicine 3: 137–139.

13. Amering M. 2010. Trialog: An Exercise in Communication between Consumers, Carers, and Professional Mental Health Workers beyond Role Stereotype. In: Conceptual Explorations on Person-Centered Medicine. International Journal of Integrated Care 10: (Suppl 10).

14. Botbol M, Lecic-Tosevski D. 2013. Person-Centered Medicine and Subjectivity. In: Jeffrey HD Cornelius-White, Renate Motschnig-Pitrik, Michael Lux (Eds). Interdisciplinary Applications of the Person-Centered Approach, Springer, New York, pp. 73–82.

15. Lebovici S. 1999. L'arbre de vie – éléments de la psychopathologie du bébé [The Tree of Life – Principles of Infant Psychopathology], Eres, Toulouse.

16. Hochmann J. 2012. Une histoire de l'empathie [A History of Empathy], Odile Jacob, Paris.

17. Ricoeur P. 1983. Temps et récit [Time and Narrative], Le Seuil, Paris.

18. Kleinman A. 1988. The Illness Narratives, Basic Books: New York.

19. Mezzich JE, Berganza CE, von Cranach M, Jorge MR, Kastrup MC, Murthy RC, Okasha A, Pull C, Sartorius N, Skodol AE, Zaudig M. 2003. Essentials of the WPA International Guidelines for Diagnostic Assessment (IGDA). British Journal of Psychiatry 182 (Suppl. 45).
20. Asociación Psiquiátrica de América Latina. 2004. Guía Latinoamericana de Diagnóstico Psiquiátrico. Guadalajara: Asociación Psiquiátrica de América Latina, Sección de Diagnóstico y Clasificación.
21. Mezzich JE, Salloum IM, Cloninger CR, Salvador-Carulla L, Kirmayer L, Banzato CE, Wallcraft J, Botbol M. 2010. Person-Centered Integrative Diagnosis: Conceptual Bases and Structural Model. Canadian Journal of Psychiatry 55: 701–708.
22. Laín-Entralgo P. 1982. El Diagnóstico Médico: Historia y Teoría, Salvat, Barcelona.
23. Schaffner KF. 2009. The Validity of Psychiatric Diagnosis: Etiopathogenic and Clinical Approaches. In: IM Salloum & JE Mezzich (Eds). Psychiatric Diagnosis: Challenges and Prospects, Wiley-Blackwell, Chichester, UK.
24. American Psychiatric Association. 2013. Diagnostic and Statistical Manual of Mental Disorders, Fifth Edition (DSM-5). Author, Arlington, VA.
25. Salloum IM, Mezzich JE. 2011. Conceptual Appraisal of the Person-Centered Integrative Diagnosis Model. International Journal of Person Centered Medicine 1: 39–42.
26. Asociación Psiquiátrica de América Latina. 2012. Guía Latinoamericana de Diagnóstico Psiquiátrico, Versión Revisada (GLADP-VR). Lima: Asociación Psiquiátrica de América Latina, Sección de Diagnóstico y Clasificación.
27. Adams N. 2012. Finding Common Ground: The Role of Integrative Diagnosis and Treatment Planning as a Pathway to Person-Centered Care. International Journal of Person Centered Medicine 2: 173–178.
28. Arora NK, McHorney CA. 2000. Patient Preferences for Medical Decision Making: Who Really Wants to Participate? Medical Care 38 (3): 335–341.
29. Mezzich JE, Botbol M, Christodoulou GN, Cloninger CR, Salloum IM (Eds). 2016. Person Centered Psychiatry, Springer, Switzerland.
30. Mezzich JE, Appleyard J, Botbol M, Ghebrehiwet T, Groves J, Salloum IM, Van Dulmen S. 2013. Ethics in Person Centered Medicine: Conceptual Place and Ongoing Developments. International Journal of Person Centered Medicine 3: 255–257.
31. Kirmayer LJ, Bennegadi R, Kastrup MC. 2016. Cultural Awareness and Responsiveness. In: JE Mezzich, M Botbol,GN Christodoulou, CR Cloninger, & IM Salloum (Eds). Person Centered Psychiatry, Heidelberg: Springer Verlag.
32. Mezzich JE. 2012. Towards a Health Experience Formulation for

Person-Centered Integrative Diagnosis. International Journal of Person Centered Medicine 2: 188–192.

33. Deegan P. 2010. A Web Application to Support Recovery and Shared Decision Making in Psychiatric Medication Clinics. Psychiatric Rehabilitation Journal 34 (1): 23–28.

34. Davidson L, Tondora J, Lawless MS, Rowe M, O'Connell MJ. 2009. A Practical Guide to Recovery Oriented Practice: Tools for Transforming Mental Health Care, Oxford Press, New York.

35. Harari YN. 2014. Sapiens. De animales a diose: Una breve historia de la humanidad. ISBN 9788499924212

36. Mezzich JE. 2007. The Dialogal Bases of Our Profession: Psychiatry with the Person. World Psychiatry 6: 129–130.

37. Peruvian Association of Person Centered Medicine and Latin American Association of Person Centered Medicine. This issue. 2018 Lima Declaration Towards the Latin American Construction of Persons-Centered Integral Health Care. International Journal of Person Centered Medicine 8(4): 11–13.

38. Saavedra JE, Otero A, Brítez J, Velásquez E, Salloum IM, Zevallos S, Luna Y, Paz V, Mezzich JE. 2017. Evaluation of the Applicability and Usefulness of the Latin American Guide for Psychiatric Diagnosis, Revised Version, in Comparison with Other International Systems among Latin American Psychiatrists. International Journal of Person Centered Medicine 7: 216–224.

PERSON-CENTERED INTEGRATIVE DIAGNOSIS: CONCEPTS AND PROCEDURES

Ihsan M. Salloum, MD, MPH[a] and Juan E. Mezzich, MD, MA, MSc, PhD[b]

ABSTRACT

The person-centered integrative diagnosis (PID) is a model that aims at putting into practice the vision of person-centered medicine affirming the whole person of the patient in context as the center of clinical care and health promotion at the individual and community levels. The PID is a novel model of conceptualizing the process and formulation of clinical diagnosis. The PID presents a paradigm shift with a broader and deeper notion of diagnosis, beyond the restricted concept of nosological diagnoses. It involves a multilevel formulation of health status (both ill and positive aspects of health) through interactive participation and engagement of clinicians, patients, and families using all relevant descriptive tools (categorization, dimensions, and narratives). The current organizational schema of the PID comprises a multilevel standardized component model integrating three main domains. Each level or major domain addresses both ill health and positive aspects of health. The first level is the assessment of health status (ill health and positive aspects of health or well-being). The second level includes contributors to health, both risk factors and protective factors. The third major level includes health experience and values. Experience with the PID through a practical guide in Latin America supported the usefulness and adequacy of the PID model.

Keywords: person-centered medicine, Person-Centered Integrative Diagnosis Model, health status, contributors to health, narratives, positive aspects of health, well-being

Corresponding Address: Professor & Inaugural Chair, Department of Neuroscience Director, Institute for Neuroscience School of Medicine HCEBL-Ste. 2.136.26 2102 Treasure Hills Blvd Harlingen, TX 78550, USA

E-mail: ihsan.salloum@utrgv.edu

---

[a] *Board Director, International College of Person Centered Medicine; Professor & Inaugural Chair, Department of Neuroscience, Director, Institute for Neuroscience University of Texas Rio Grande Valley School of Medicine; Chair, Section on Classification, Diagnostic Assessment & Nomenclature; Emeritus Professor of Psychiatry, University of Miami Miller School of Medicine.*
[b] *Professor of Psychiatry, Icahn School of Medicine at Mount Sinai, New York; Secretary General and Former President, International College of Person Centered Medicine; Council Member and Former President, World Psychiatric Association*

INTRODUCTION

Person-centered medicine (PCM) embraces holistic concepts of health advocating the whole person in context as the center and goal of clinical care and public health [1]. PCM strives toward a personalized approach to care within an integrated biological, psychological, social, and cultural framework. Ancient traditions as well as modern concepts of care highlight the holistic concept of health [2–9]. This is also reflected in the World Health Organization's definition of health as not merely the absence of disease but a state of "complete physical, emotional, and social well-being" [10].

The overarching principles of PCM gleaned from a reiterative process involving comprehensive literature reviews, focus groups, and international expert consensus [11] include the following:

1. Ethical Commitment, which refers to respect for the dignity of every person involved in the care process (patients, family, clinicians), respect for the patient's rights, promoting the patient's autonomy and empowerment, paying attention to the patient's personal values, choices, and needs, and the fulfillment of the patient's life project.
2. Cultural Sensitivity "this refers to cultural Awareness and responsiveness," of "being attentive to the patient's ethnic identity, cultural values, spiritual needs, language, communication needs and preferences, and the patient's gender identity and sexual needs."
3. Holistic Approach with a bio-psycho-socio-cultural-spiritual framework and equal attention to both ill health (diseases, disabilities) and positive health or well-being (functioning, resilience, resources, and quality of life).
4. Relational Focus, establishing therapeutic alliance and cultivating the clinician–patient relationship, displaying empathy in the care process, and establishing trust during clinical communication and care.
5. Individualization of Care with focus on the patient's uniqueness, promoting the patient's personal growth and development, considering the patient's personal choices in life and social context.
6. Shared Understanding and Shared Decision-making promoting shared understanding of patient's health situation, conducting a diagnosis of health (rather than just ill health) and shared decision making for treatment planning and the care process.
7. People-Centered Organization of Services including advocacy for the health and rights of all people in the community, people's participation in the planning of health services, promoting partnership at all levels of service organization, promoting quality and excellence in personalized services,

service responsiveness to community needs and expectations, and integration and coordination of services around patients' needs. It also includes emphasis on people-centered primary care services to ensure continuity of care, and services informed by international perspectives and developments for person-centered care.

8. Person-Centered Education, Training and Research with a health system committed to promoting person-centered public health education, person-centered health professional training, and person-centered clinical research.

The process of diagnosis is central to health care practices and to implementing the goals and principles of care. However, traditional diagnostic approaches are focused almost entirely on identifying ill health and have paid limited attention to the totality of health, with scant consideration of positive aspects of health.

The Person-Centered Integrative Diagnosis model (PID) is a key diagnostic tool of person-centered medicine. It operationalizes principles of medicine for the person into an integrated individualized diagnostic model applicable to regular clinical care [12]. The development of this model initiated under the auspices of the World Psychiatric Association's Institutional Program on Psychiatry for the Person (WPA General Assembly, 2005). The PID embodies the principles of PCM and their application in regular clinical care and is adaptable to the diverse clinical realities and needs. Importantly, it is measurable, employing categorical, dimensional and narrative approaches allowing for quantitative, qualitative, and mixed analysis to assess the impact of the application of this model on the processes of care as well as on patients' outcome.

Thus, the PID aims at putting into practice the vision of person-centered medicine affirming the whole person of the patient in context as the center of clinical care and health promotion at the individual and community levels. The purposes of the Person-Centered Integrative Diagnosis (PID) model are to provide a diagnosis of health status (ill & positive health), to serve as informational bases for clinical care and public health, to enhance clinical care and outcome, to promote recovery and health restoration, and to promote prevention and health promotion. Thus, the PID is viewed to be a diagnostic model *of the person* (of the totality of the person's health, ill, and positive), *by the person* (including clinicians considered as full human beings and not merely "undescript technicians"), *for the person* (for the fulfillment of the person's health & life project), and *with the person* (in a respectful and empowering relationship).

In the following section we discuss key paradigm shifts introduced by the Person-Centered Diagnostic Model (PID), and will present its structure as an integrated, personalized, multilevel assessment of health status.

KEY PARADIGM SHIFTS OF THE PERSON-CENTERED INTEGRATIVE DIAGNOSIS (PID) MODEL

The first key paradigm shift involves the essential notion of diagnosis. The PID broadens the traditional notion of "diagnosis" from a restrictive nosological understanding to a broader and deeper notion of diagnosis to include the totality of health encompassing both its positive and ill aspects. This encompassing notion of diagnosis is in concordance with the WHO's 1946 visionary definition of health mentioned earlier and it is well captured by the 20th-century Spanish philosopher and humanist, Ortega y Gasset' (1883–1955) statement "I am I and my circumstance" [13], which embodies the PCM and PID's vision of considering "the whole person in context" as the center and goal of clinical care and public health. Furthermore, the PID promotes a notion of diagnosis as a process involving the interactive participation and engagement of clinicians, patients, and families, leading to the formulation and articulation of the patient's health in its totality.

The primary role of diagnosis in medicine as the basic unit in the process of medical care is indicated by its multiple functions. Diagnosis is essential for communication among health professionals and other stakeholders, it is central for the process of clinical care and the identification and treatment of disorders, it is important for prevention and health promotion, and it is necessary for conducting research, testing interventions and understanding disease mechanisms. Furthermore, diagnosis is needed for education and training and for a host of administrative purposes from quality improvement to reimbursement activities. Feinstein [14] cogently expressed the pivotal role of diagnosis in the clinicians' work "Diagnostic categories provide the locations where clinicians store the observations of clinical experience" and "The diagnostic taxonomy establishes the patterns, according to which clinicians observe, think, remember and act."

The PID's broader notion of diagnosis with the focus on the totality of health and on giving substantial attention to positive aspects of health as well as diagnosis as an interactive process helps to enhance the positive connotations associated with diagnosis. These include increased understanding and empowerment. This approach also contributes to mitigating negative connotations such as pejorative value judgments, stigma, and labeling associated with certain diagnosis (e.g., psychiatric conditions).

The second key feature of the PID is its partnership approach with an emphasis on an inclusive and collaborative process. All stakeholders in the clinical encounter are empowered as protagonists of the diagnostic process. The diagnostic formulation is an ongoing process, constructed through interactive partnership involving a dialogue among the primary stakeholders and evaluators. The PID upholds the dignity, values, and aspirations of the person seeking care through a partnership of equals that includes the clinician (the conventional expert), the patient (the protagonist, informationally and ethically), the family (crucial support group), and community members (teachers, social workers, etc.). This partnership approach enhances self-efficacy, which has been found to mediate positive health and healing [15].

The third paradigm shift is the inclusion of narrative and subjective experience into the diagnostic model. The narrative reflects the uniqueness of the person's health experience as well as other stakeholders' subjective experience into the diagnostic process. The narrative corresponds to the idiographic personalized content that captures the experience of illness. This includes topics such as suffering, values, meaning of illness, expectation of health, and the cultural experience of illness and care. It also includes the experience of well-being such as personal belonging and uniqueness as well as cultural identity. Beliefs about health and illness are crucial for self-care and may influence behavioral and physiological responses to illness [16–17].

THE MULTILEVEL SCHEME OF THE PERSON-CENTERED INTEGRATIVE DIAGNOSIS MODEL

The initial development of the PID model was anchored within the well-established experience of the World Psychiatric Association in the development of diagnostic models and contributions to the central issue of international diagnoses in psychiatry [18–21]. The current organizational schema of the PID comprises a multilevel standardized component model integrating three main domains. Each level or major domain addresses both ill health and positive aspects of health [21].

The first major level is the assessment of the health status (ill health and positive aspects of health or well-being), the second major level includes contributors to the health status. These are contributors to ill health and contributors to well-being. The third major level includes health experiences and values (of ill health and of well-being). Each of these levels is further organized into key domains. See Figure 1 corresponding to the Diagnostic Formulation of the Latin American Guide for Psychiatric Diagnosis, Revised Version (GLADP-VR) [22, 23].

The health status levels document the illness and its burden. Disorders, as classified in the WHO International Classification of Diseases, Revision 10 (ICD-10), are documented under this domain. Functioning (or disabilities) is also considered under these domains. Overall functioning, as well as major areas of functioning related to personal care, occupational functioning, functioning with family, and social functioning are considered and rated on a 0 to 10 Likert scale, as is done for well-being. A narrative component complements the assessment of this level, where patients and clinicians can provide a narrative, personalized account of this level of assessment.

Name: _____ Code: _____ Date: _____

Age: _____ Sex: M/F Marital Status: _____ Occupation: _____

I. HEALTH STATUS

Clinical Disorders and Related Conditions (as classified in CIE-10).

A. Mental Disorders (in general, including personality and developmental disorders, and related conditions):

	Codes:

B. General Medical Conditions:

	Codes:

Functioning of the Person (Use the following scale to evaluate each of the functioning areas)

Poorest	Minimal	Marginal	Acceptable	Substantial	Excellent
0 1	2 3	4 5	6 7	8 9	10

Functioning Areas		Score						
A	Personal care	0	2	4	6	8	10	?
B	Occupational (wage earner, student, etc.)	0	2	4	6	8	10	?
C	With family	0	2	4	6	8	10	?
D	Social in general	0	2	4	6	8	10	?

Degree of Well-being (Indicate level perceived by the person on the following scale, optionally using a suitable instrument).

Poorest										Excellent
0	1	2	3	4	5	6	7	8	9	10

II. HEALTH CONTRIBUTING FACTORS

Risk Factors: [] Abnormal weight [] Hyper-cholesterolemia [] Hyperglicemia [] Hypertensión [] Tabacco [] Alcohol [] Family psychiatric problems [] Severe child trauma [] Prolongued or severe stress

Additional information: _____

Protective Factors: [] Healthy diet [] Physical activity [] Creative activities [] Social participation

Additional information: _____

III. HEALTH EXPERIENCES AND EXPECTATIONS

Personal and cultural identity: _____
_____

Suffering (its recognition, idioms of distress, illness beliefs): _____
_____

Experiences and expectations on health care: _____
_____

Figure 1. GLADP-VR Personalized Diagnostic Formulation Form

The contributors to health level addresses both intrinsic and extrinsic contributors to the health status utilizing a bio-psycho-social framework. This level also documents specific contributors to ill health derived from the World Health Professions Alliance health improvement cards [24]. Specifically listed health promoters include diet, physical activity, creative activity, social involvement, and others. Specific health risk includes overweight, high lipid, high glucose, high blood pressure, alcohol and tobacco use, family history, early life trauma, significant stress, and others. This level also includes a narrative component.

The third level corresponds to the idiographic personalized narrative capturing health experience and values. It includes experience of well-being including personal values and cultural identity and experience of ill health to include suffering, meaning of illness, values, and cultural experience of illness and care and expectation of health care.

The PID schema and its GLADP-VR practical application are aimed at forming the informational bases for intervention and care, such as developing treatment plans to guide recovery and health restoration, as well as to providing the informational bases for education, public health planning and for administrative functions.

The PID avails all relevant descriptive tools, including categorical, dimensional, and narrative approaches. These approaches allow for capturing quantitative and categorical assignments above a certain threshold. The use of narrative offers the possibility of a deeper and richer personalized description of a relevant domain.

The PID model was officially adopted by the Latin American Guide to Psychiatric Diagnosis (GLADP-VR) [23], through which significant experience was gained in the application of the PID in regular patient care. Experience with the GLADP documented the effectiveness of the PID model in providing a personalized diagnostic formulation and in addressing cultural issues [25].

CONCLUSIONS

The person-centered integrative diagnosis (PID) aims at putting into practice the vision of person-centered medicine affirming the whole person of the patient in context as the center of clinical care and health promotion at individual and community levels. The PID is a novel model of conceptualizing the process and formulation of clinical diagnosis. The PID presents several paradigm shifts with a broader and deeper notion of diagnosis of the whole of health, beyond the more restricted conceptualization of nosological diagnoses. It involves a multilevel formulation of health (both ill and positive aspects of health), arrived at through interactive participation and engagement of clinicians, patients, and families using various relevant descriptive tools (categorization, dimensions, and narratives). Extensive experience with the PID model through its GLADP-VR practical application demonstrated its utility and practicality of use within regular clinical care in providing a personalized and culturally informative diagnosis within a partnership framework that actively engages the patient into the diagnostic and care process.

ACKNOWLEDGMENTS AND DISCLOSURES

The authors do not report any conflicts of interest.

REFERENCES

1. Mezzich JE. 2007. Psychiatry for the Person: Articulating Medicine's Science and Humanism. World Psychiatry 6 (2): 1–3.
2. Herrman H, Saxena S, Moodie R. 2005. Promoting Mental Health: Concepts, Emerging Evidence, Practice, WHO, Geneva.
3. World Health Organization. 1999.WHO's New Global Strategies for Mental Health. Factsheet 217.
4. U.S. Presidential Commission on Mental Health. 2003. Achieving the Promise: Transforming Mental Health Care in America. Final Report. DHHS Pub N: SMA-03-3832. Rockville, Maryland: Department of Health and Human Services.
5. World Health Organization European Ministerial Conference on Mental Health. Mental Health Action Plan for Europe: Facing the Challenges, Building Solutions. Helsinki, Finland, January 12–15, 2005. EUR/04/5047810/7.
6. Patwardhan B, Warude D, Pushpangadan P, Bhatt N. 2005. Ayurveda and Traditional Chinese Medicine: A Comparative Overview. Evidence-Based Complementary and Alternative Medicine 2: 465–473.
7. Christodoulou GN. (Ed) 1987. Psychosomatic Medicine, Plenum Press, New York.
8. Anthony W. 1993. Recovery from Mental Illness. The Guiding Vision of the Mental Health Service Systems in the 1990s. Psychosocial Rehabilitation Journal 16: 11–23.
9. Amering M, Schmolke M. 2007. Recovery – Das Ende der Unheilbarkeit, Psychiatrie-Verlag, Bonn.
10. World Health Organization. 1946. WHO Constitution, WHO, Geneva.
11. Mezzich JE, Kirisci L, Salloum IM, Trivedi JK, Kar SK, Adams N, Wallcraft J. 2016. Systematic Conceptualization of Person Centered Medicine and Development and Validation of a Measurement Index. International Journal of Person Centered Medicine 6 (4): 219–247.
12. Mezzich JE, Salloum IM. 2009. Towards a Person-Centered Integrative Diagnosis. In: IM Salloum & JE Mezzich (Eds). Psychiatric Diagnosis: Context and Prospects, Wiley-Blackwell, Oxford, UK, pp. 297–302.

13. Lain-Entralgo P. 1982. El Diagnostico Medico: Historia y Teoría, Salvat, Barcelona.
14. Feinstein AR. 1967. Clinical Judgment, Robert E. Krieger, Huntington, NY.
15. Mezzich JE. This issue. Setting a Common Ground for Collaborative Care and Clinical Interviewing: International Journal of Person Centered Medicine 8(3): 29–40.
16. Kirmayer L, Mezzich JE, Van Staden W. 2016. Health Experience and Values. In: JE Mezzich, M Botbol, GN Christodoulou, CR Cloninger, & Salloum IM (Eds). Person Centered Psychiatry, Springer, Switzerland, pp. 179–199.
17. Mezzich JE. 2012. Towards a Health Experience Formulation for Person-Centered Integrative Diagnosis. International Journal of Person Centered Medicine 2: 188–192.
18. Mezzich JE, Ustun TB. 2002. International Classification and Diagnosis: Critical Experience and Future Directions. Psychopathology 35 (Special Issue): 55–202.
19. Banzato CEM, Mezzich JE, Berganza CE. (Eds) 2005. Philosophical and Methodological Foundations of Psychiatric Diagnosis. Psychopathology 38 (Special Issue Jul–Aug).
20. World Psychiatric Association. 2003. Essentials of the World Psychiatric Association's International Guidelines for Diagnostic Assessment (IGDA). British Journal of Psychiatry 182 (Suppl 45): s37–s66.
21. Mezzich JE, Salloum IM, Cloninger CR, Salvador-Carulla L, Kirmayer L, Banzato CE, Wallcraft J, Botbol M. 2010. Person-Centered Integrative Diagnosis: Conceptual Bases and Structural Model. Canadian Journal of Psychiatry 55: 701–708.
22. Mezzich JE, Otero A, Saavedra JE, Salloum IM. 2013. The GLADP-VR Person-Centered Diagnostic Formulation: Background, Concepts, and Structure. International Journal of Person Centered Medicine 3: 228–242.
23. Asociación Psiquiátrica de América Latina (APAL). 2012. Guia Latinoamericana de Diagnostico Psiquiátrico, Versión Revisada (GLADP-VR) (Latin American Guide of Psychiatric Diagnosis, Revised Version). Lima: APAL.
24. WHPA Health Improvement Card: https://www.whpa.org/sites/default/files/2018-12/ncd_Health-Improvement-Card_web.pdf
25. Saavedra JE, Otero A, Brítez J, Velásquez E, Salloum IM, Zevallos S, Luna Y, Paz V, Mezzich JE. 2017. Evaluation of the Applicability and Usefulness of the Latin American Guide for Psychiatric Diagnosis, Revised Version, in Comparison with Other International Systems among Latin American Psychiatrists. International Journal of Person Centered Medicine7: 216–224.

CONTINUITY AND INTEGRATION OF PERSON-CENTERED ASSESSMENT AND CARE ACROSS THE LIFE CYCLE

W. James Appleyard, MD[a] and Michel Botbol, MD, MSc[b]

ABSTRACT

Health is a consequence of multiple determinants operating in interrelated genetic, biological, behavioral, social, and economic contexts that change as a person develops.

The timing and sequence of such events and experiences influence the health and development of both individuals and populations. A life course perspective offers a more joined up approach with significant implications for long term health gain. A three-dimensional picture needs to evolve laterally in the present, longitudinally from earlier life events and likely future projections, and vertically from the advances in the medical sciences.

Keywords: attunement, biopsychosocial, adverse child event, allostatic, empathy, cumulative and programming events

Correspondence Address: Prof. W. James Appleyard, Thimble Hall Blean Common, Kent CT2 9JJ, United Kingdom

E-mail: jimappleyard2510@aol.com

INTRODUCTION

The health and well-being of a person are complex adaptive processes related to the consequences of genetic, biological, social, cultural, behavioral, and economic determinants throughout the life course [1]. Circumstances change as the person

---

[a] *Board Advisor and Former President, International College of Person Centered Medicine; Former President, World Medical Association; Former President, International Association of Medical Colleges*
[b] *Board Director, International College of Person-Centered Medicine; Secretary for Scientific Publications, World Psychiatric Association; Emeritus Professor of Child and Adolescent Psychiatry, University of Western Brittany, Brest, France*

develops with accumulative risk and protective factors especially during critical and sensitive periods in the early years.

Specific alterations in interactions between genes and environment and disturbances in homeostatic equilibrium and dysregulation due to stress are now being linked to the development of health disorders like cardiovascular disease, hypertension, cancer, and cognitive decline [2]. A life course perspective offers a more joined up approach with significant implications for long-term health gain. There is an emphasis on an integrated continuum of early intervention and education rather than of disconnected and unrelated stages. Each stage in the life of a person exerts influence on the next.

Disparities in health outcomes and in the psychosocial factors contributing to them are present early in life and are expressed and compounded during a person's lifetime. Risk factors are embedded in a person's biological makeup, manifested in the disparities in a population's health, and maintained by social, cultural, and economic forces. Research on health disparities has demonstrated the effect of many determinants interacting in various contexts at developmentally sensitive points.

Understanding the well-established links between events in the early part of the life course and their inherent biopsychosocial implications with the maintenance of health and the onset of disorders and disease later in life is essential for planning a person- and people-centered approach to the health care of the individual and to preventive strategies effective for each community and large populations [3]. A three-dimensional picture needs to evolve laterally in the present, longitudinally from earlier life events and likely future projections, and vertically from the advances in the medical sciences.

LONGITUDINAL STUDIES

The Adverse Childhood Event (ACE) study [5] provides retrospective and prospective analysis covering 17,000 privately insured middle-class Americans of the effect of early traumatic life experience on later well-being, social function, health risks, disease burden, health care costs, and life expectancy. An individual's current state of health and well-being was matched retrospectively approximately 50 years after adverse events in childhood, and then the cohort was followed forward to match the Adverse Childhood Event (ACE) score prospectively against doctor office visits, emergency room visits, hospitalization, pharmacy costs, and death.

Each participant was assigned an individual ACE score, which was a count of the number of categories of adverse childhood experience encountered in their first 18 years. These are (1) emotional abuse, (2) physical abuse, (3) contact sexual abuse, (4) mother treated violently, (5) household member an alcoholic or drug user, (6) household member in prison, (7) household member chronically depressed, suicidal, mentally ill, or in psychiatric hospital, (8) subject not being raised by both biological parents, (9) physical neglect, and (10) emotional neglect.

The findings were stark. A study participant found to score 1 on the adverse childhood experience score had an 87% probability of more such experiences. One in six people had scores of 4 or above. It was found that there is a strong relationship between ACE score and self-acknowledged chronic depression and later suicide attempts. It appears that depression is common and has deep roots, usually going back to the developmental years of life. The higher the ACE score the greater the likelihood of later smoking, alcoholism, intravenous drug use, obesity, and high-level promiscuity.

The authors of the study conclude that "all told, it is clear that adverse childhood experiences have a profound, proportionate, and long-lasting effect on well-being," whether this is measured by depression or suicide attempts, by protective unconscious devices like overeating and even amnesia or by what they refer to as "self-help attempts," the use of street drugs or alcohol to modulate feelings.

They argue that the study points to a credible basis for a new paradigm of primary care medical practice and advocate that treatment should begin with a comprehensive biopsychosocial evaluation of all patients. After such an evaluation was administered to 200,000 patients, there was a 35% reduction in visits to doctors' offices during the following year.

The work of David Barker and his colleagues pointed to the importance of early life factors in the programming of risk for chronic disease in adults during critical periods [2]. Using historical cohort designs, Barker's group analyzed birth weight data and measures of development in the first years of life and found extensive evidence that adult somatic response patterns were programmed in early life. Birth weight, placenta size, and weight gain and growth in the first year of life were found to be associated with cardiovascular disease, diabetes, and hypertension in the fifth and sixth decades [3].

Specific alterations in interactions between genes and environment and disturbances in homeostatic equilibrium and dysregulation due to stress are now being linked to the development of health disorders like cardiovascular disease, hypertension, cancer, and cognitive decline [4].

The ability to achieve stability through change (allostasis) hypothesizes a connection between an individual's psychosocial environment to diseases and functional declines by way of dysregulation in various neuroendocrine systems. Examples of the adaptive price of stress-induced wear and tear ("weathering") on the organism include pushing the endocrine system toward diabetes, or the cardiovascular system toward coronary artery disease and hypertension.

EMPATHY

Attunement takes place when the parent and child are emotionally functioning in tune with each other and where the child's emotional needs for love, acceptance, and security are met. Without satisfactory early attunement to the primary caregiver, the development of empathy can be greatly impaired. Empathy entails the ability to step outside oneself emotionally and be able to suppress temporarily one's own perspective on events to take another's. It is present when the observed experiences of others come to affect our own thoughts and feelings in a caring fashion. When a parent consistently fails to show any empathy with the child's expression of particular emotions, the child can drop those emotions from his or her repertoire. Empathy is also perceived as a prime requirement for a citizen to be of the law-abiding "self-regulator" type.

Because the infant's cortical and hippocampal emotional circuits require significant time and experience to mature, the child must regulate its inner world primarily through attachment relationships with primary caregivers. Babies who are healthily attached to their carer can regulate their emotions as they mature because the cortex, which exercises rational thought and control, has developed properly. However, when early conditions result in underdevelopment of the cortex, the child lacks an "emotional guardian."[5]

As Shore [6] concluded: "The child's first relationship," the one with the mother, acts as a template that permanently moulds the individual's capacity to enter into all later emotional relationships". Small children look to a parent's facial expressions and other non-verbal signals to determine how to respond and feel in a strange or ambiguous situation. The same type of mechanisms has been also found to be crucial for the transgenerational transmission of attachment patterns and the intersubjective development at large [7] through the role of early microbehaviors [8].

It is well documented that infants can perceive and remember maternal microbehaviors and tend to imitate the facial expressions they observe in others. These properties could be of crucial importance for the construction of the infant's self and the development of his subjectivity and intersubjectivity through early sensory-motor experiences. Furthermore, the recent discovery of the Mirror Neuron System (MNS) has led to new perspectives regarding the neurobiological substratum for intersubjectivity. Several studies favor the hypothesis that by neurologically "simulating" other individuals' actions, this system does not simply involve the observation of actions but makes it possible to access the mental states of the individual being observed by another and, more particularly, his intentions.

Such simulation is automatic and involuntary and needs no conscious thought regarding the meaning of the action or the mental state of the individual whose acts are being observed. Could the MNS be the anatomical substratum for any transmission and particularly those of adverse experiences? Following this hypothesis, these behaviors would have an intermediary role between the mother's and the child's unconscious representations, influencing the quality of the child's subjective and intersubjective development. "One possible function [of MNS] could be to promote learning by imitation. When new motor skills are learned, one often spends the first training phases trying to replicate the movements of an observed instructor. The MNS could in principle facilitate that kind of learning" [9].

Far fewer girls than boys show conduct disorder by age 21, but of those who did, 30% of the "at risk" conduct-disordered girls, had become teenage mothers, whereas there had been not a single teenage birth to the conduct-disordered girls from the not-at-risk group. Of those "conduct-disordered and at risk" teenage mothers, 43% were in abusive, violent relationships, having found their partners from within the "at risk" boys. Subsequent follow-up at age 26 showed the pattern was maintained. Immature mothers with no strong parenting skills and violent partners had already given birth to the next generation of "at risk" children [10]. The quality of parents' interaction with their babies and young children is known to influence children's expectations about relationships not only during childhood but also in later years [11].

Another example of the long-term effects of impaired early relationships on children's long-term development is the effect of maternal depression on infant development. Relative to control mothers, depressed mothers express less positive and more negative affect, are less attentive and engaged with their infants, and, when engaged, are more intrusive and controlling and fail to respond adaptively to their infants' emotional signals [12].

Their infants have shorter attention spans, less motivation to master tasks, elevated heart rates, elevated cortisol levels, and reduced EEG activity in the right frontal cortex, all of which correlate with the experience of negative affect in adults. Longitudinal data on infants of depressed mothers indicate that elevated heart rates and cortisol can persist.

RISK AND PROTECTIVE FACTORS INFLUENCING THE LIFE COURSE

Health development can be understood as the interaction between *cumulative* and *programming* mechanisms, which are controlled by genes, experiences, and past adaptive responses along the life course.

Cumulative mechanisms are dose or exposure dependent. They are based on the relationship between the number of social risk factors that a child experiences and his or her intellectual attainment [13] or on the cumulative effects on various outcomes from a lifelong exposure to a specific risk factor such as cigarette smoking. *Programming mechanisms* refer to the strong, independent effect of risks, exposures, and adaptive responses during sensitive or critical developmental periods, many of which occur early in life. The range and extent of programming effects of biological and psychophysiological processes influence long-term health development [14].

Critical or "sensitive" periods are those stages of functional development when a regulatory pathway is being constructed or modified and the developing organism is particularly responsive and sensitive to favorable or unfavorable environmental factors. A critical period when a developmental path is determined, a sensitive period of development, is a time when a favorable or unfavorable exposure has a stronger effect than it would have at other times.

When an early environmental stimulus or insult occurs during a critical or sensitive period, it programs a long-term or permanent change in an organism's functional system [15]. Hormones, antigens, and drugs all can serve as programming agents that deactivate, activate, or alter functional pathways. Programmed long-term adaptations are the result of interactions between genes and the environment in which environmental factors influence and help set the operating parameters of specific genes during critical and sensitive developmental periods. Studies of the structure and function of the visual area of the cerebral cortex in primates show that the establishment of neural connections and their subsequent pruning depend on the type of visual stimulation provided by the environment [16].

THE NEED FOR A NEW PERSPECTIVE ON HEALTH CARE

The implication of the developmental features over the life course with a particular emphasis on the early years calls for a framework for the provision of health care that offers a radically different conceptualization of individual and population health. Assessment of the health status of both individuals and populations need to understand the inherent bio-psycho-social potential and differences even in the apparently "healthy." These differences result in varying levels of resilience that have profound implications for future health status and development in the face of risks and adversity.

Currently, the health of individuals and populations is measured according to health outcomes – disease, disability, dysfunction, and mortality. The most widely used measures of health are based on deficits, using levels of decline to define health status [17]. Even relatively integrative parameters like the health-related quality of life (HRQL) include instruments that focus on the extent of declines from a hypothetical state of "full health."

Differences in developmental life course projections are likely to explain much of the variance in the nature and rate of later declines in health. A person-centered approach not only measures an individual's illness but also focuses on health and well-being. Measuring positive health supports health policies based on building both individual and community health, a concept illustrated in the field of community development [18], which encourages the use of positive health measurements that identify positive health and well-being and not merely disease and deficits [19].

The current management approaches involving additive health care systems based increasingly on vertical management are not designed to reflect the needs of individuals. Such systems can be reduced to their component parts and oftentimes two or three of these elements, viewed as being the most significant, are focused upon at the expense of several other related factors influencing the health of the individual person or community.

Complex adaptive systems however are composed of many components that reciprocally influence one another, so that they behave more like biological systems than the mechanical deterministic additive systems of separate parts. Complex adaptive systems provide an important model for understanding difficult problems involving many interacting adaptive agents, such as managing health care systems, understanding economic markets, encouraging innovation in dynamic economies, providing for sustainable human growth, preserving ecosystems, and promoting health [20–21].

CONCLUSIONS

Understanding the well-established links between events in the early part of the life course and their inherent biopsychosocial implications with the maintenance of health and the onset of disorders and disease later in life is essential for planning a person- and people-centered approach to the heath care of the individual and to preventive strategies effective for each community and large populations. A three-dimensional picture needs to evolve laterally in the present, longitudinally from earlier life events and likely future projections, and vertically from the advances in the medical sciences. From these perspectives, integrated person-centered proposals should emerge within a responsible ethical framework respecting each individual and placing their well-being and their welfare as the first consideration. We need an integrated conceptual approach to translate this knowledge into effective health and social care.

ACKNOWLEDGMENTS AND DISCLOSURES

The authors do not report any conflicts of interest.

REFERENCES

1. Appleyard J. 2015. Person-Centered and Integrated Care across the Life-Cycle. International Journal of Person Centered Medicine 5 (1): 15–20.
2. Barker DJP. 1998. Mothers, Babies, and Health in Later Life, Churchill Livingstone, Edinburgh.
3. Martyn CN, Barker DJP, Osmond C. 1996. Mothers' Pelvic Size, Fetal Growth, and Coronary Heart Disease in Men in the UK. Lancet 348: 1264–1268.
4. McEwen BS. 1998. Stress, Adaptation, and Disease: Allostasis and Allostatic Load. Annals of the New York Academy of Sciences 840: 33–44.
5. Felitti V, Anda RF. 2010. The Relationship of Adverse Childhood Experiences to Adult Health, Wellbeing, Social Function and Healthcare. In: R Lanius & E Vermetten (Eds). The Hidden Epidemic: The Impact of Early Life Trauma on Health and Disease, Cambridge, UK: Cambridge University Press, 2010.
6. Shore R. 1997. Rethinking the Brain. New Insights into Early Development, Families and Work Institute, New York.
7. Botbol M. 2010. Towards an Integrative Neuroscientific and Psychodynamic Approach to the Transmission of Attachment. Journal of Physiology (Paris) 104: 263–271.
8. Peck SD. 2003. Measuring Sensitivity Moment-by-Moment: A Microanalytic Look at the Transmission of Attachment. Attachment & Human Development 5: 38–63.
9. Gallese V, Goldman A. 1998. Mirror Neurons and the Simulation Theory of Mind Reading. Trends in Cognitive Sciences 2, 493–501.
10. Bremner JD, Vythilingham M, Vermetten E, Southwick SM, McGlashen T, Nazeer A. 2003. MRI and PET Study of Deficits in Hippocampal Structure and function in Women with Childhood Sexual Abuse and Posttraumatic Stress Disorder. American Journal of Psychiatry 160: 924–932.
11. Department of Health, UK. 2008. Children and Young People in Mind: The Final Report of the National CAMHS Review, UK Department of Health, London.
12. Crittenden PM. 2011. Raising Parents: Attachment, Parenting and Child Safety, Taylor and Francis, Abingdon.

13. Powers C, Hertzman C, 1997. Social and Biological Pathways Linking Early Life and Adult Disease. British Medical Bulletin 53 (1): 210–221.
14. Leon DA. 1998. Fetal Growth and Adult Disease. European Journal of Clinical Medicine 52 (S1): S72–S82.
15. Lucas A. 1998. Programming by Early Nutrition: An Experimental Approach. Journal of Nutrition128: 401S–406S.
16. Ben-Shlomo Y, Kuh D. 2002. A Life Course Approach to Chronic Disease Epidemiology: Conceptual Models, Empirical Challenges and Interdisciplinary Perspectives. International Journal of Epidemiology 31: 285–293.
17. Young TK. 1998. Population Health: Concepts and Methods, Oxford University Press, New York.
18. McKnight JL. 1999. Two Tools for Well-being: Health Systems and Communities. Journal of Perinatology 19: S12–S15.
19. Patrick DL, Erickson P. 1993. Health Status and Health Policy: Quality of Life in Health Care Evaluation and Resource Allocation, Oxford University Press, New York.
20. Cloninger CR, Salloum IM, Mezzich JE. 2012. The Dynamic Origins of Positive Health and Wellbeing. International Journal of Person Centered Medicine 2: 1–9.
21. Wilson CR, Appleyard J, Mezzich JE, Abou-Saleh M, Gutkin C, Van Weel C, Epperly T. 2016. Challenges and Opportunities for Person Centered Integrated Care through the Life Course. International Journal of Person Centered Medicine 6: 79–82.

SECTION 3

Care Planning, Shared Decision Making and Inter-Professional Collaboration

EDITORIAL INTRODUCTION

ICPCM EDUCATIONAL PROGRAM ON PERSON-CENTERED CARE: CARE PLANNING, SHARED DECISION MAKING, AND INTERPROFESSIONAL COLLABORATION

W. James Appleyard, MA, MD, FRCP[a] and Juan E. Mezzich, MD, MA, MSc, PhD[b]

Keywords: person-centered medicine, educational program, person-centered care, International College of Person Centered Medicine, listening, narrative, communication, common ground, comorbidity, palliative care, interprofessional collaboration

Correspondence Address: Prof. W. James Appleyard, Thimble Hall Blean Common, Kent CT2 9JJ, United Kingdom

E-mail: jimappleyard2510@aol.com

INTRODUCTION

This section of the monograph includes the third part of the Educational Program on Person-Centered Care of the International College of Person Centered Medicine (ICPCM) that in its initial version was presented at the 6th International Congress of Person Centered Medicine in New Delhi in November 2018. The overall themes of the four papers [1–4] are the planning of care, shared decision making, and interprofessional collaboration. In addition, there is the Lima Declaration 2018 entitled "Towards a Latin American Construction of

---

[a] Board Advisor and Former President, International College of Person Centered Medicine; Former President, World Medical Association; President, International Association of Medical Colleges
[b] Professor of Psychiatry, Icahn School of Medicine at Mount Sinai, New York; Hipólito Unanue Chair of Person-Centered Medicine, San Marcos National University, Lima; Former President, World Psychiatric Association; Secretary General and Former President, International College of Person Centered Medicine

Persons-Centered Integral Health Care," which recognizes how important these concepts are to the development of general strategies for integrated health care with persons placed at the center of and as the goal of health actions. Reports from the Symposium on Person-Centered Medicine held during the 2018 World Medical Association's Conference in Reykjavik and the First Peruvian Conference on Person-Centered Medicine add further evidence of the importance of these perspectives.

Shared decision making has been shown to improve patients' knowledge and ability to participate in decisions about their care and improve the quality of clinical decision making. Clinicians and patients (often with family participation) decide together based on clinical evidence and the patient's informed preferences about any appropriate investigations, treatments, management, or support packages. It involves exploring relevant evidence-based information about options, outcomes, and uncertainties, together with decision support counseling and a systematic approach to recording and implementing patient's preferences [5, 6]. Though also leading to improvements in health outcomes for people with long-term health problems [7], it is only slowly filtering into mainstream clinical practice [8].

THE CLINICAL CONSULTATION

Shared decision making starts with a person's story, which should be allowed to be recounted as a complicated narrative of health and illness told in words, silences, gestures, physical observations, overlain not only by objective findings but also with associated implications, fears, and hopes. The narration is a therapeutic central act because to find the words to contain the disorder and its attendant worries gives shape to and control over the uncertainties of the illness. As the physician listens to the patient, he or she follows the narrative thread of the story in all its existential cultural, familial, biological, social, psychological, and spiritual dimensions.

This encompasses an awareness of health and disease from which the meaning and purpose in both an illness and the experience of recovery emerge. Disorder "labels" become secondary to the life of the person.

LISTENING

The act of listening, so essential to the process, enlists the physician's interior resources – memories, association curiosities, creativity, interpretive powers, and allusions to other stories by the person and others to identify meaning. Only then can the physician hear and confront the person's narrative questions "what is wrong with me?" Why is this happening to me? And what will be the result [9]?

Listening to stories of illness and recognizing that there are often no clear answers to patients' narrative questions demand the courage and generosity to tolerate and to bear witness to unfair losses and random tragedies [10]. Accomplishing such acts of witnessing allows the physician to proceed to his or her more recognizably clinical narrative tasks: to establish a therapeutic alliance, to generate and proceed through a differential diagnosis, to interpret physical findings and laboratory reports correctly, to experience and convey empathy for the patient's experience [11], and, as a result of all these, to engage the patient for effective care.

If the physician cannot perform these narrative tasks, the patient might not tell the whole story, might not ask the most frightening questions, and might not feel heard [12]. The resultant diagnostic workup might be unfocused and therefore more expensive than need be, the correct ailment might be missed, the clinical care might be marked by noncompliance and the search for another opinion, and the therapeutic relationship might be shallow and ineffective. The narrative is absorbing. It engages the listening physician and invites an interpretation. It gives him or her the experience of "living through," not simply "knowledge about" the characters and events in the story.

EFFECTIVE PRACTICE

The effective practice of medicine therefore requires narrative competence, that is, the ability to listen, acknowledge, absorb, interpret, and act on the stories and plights of other people [13]. The narrative also provides information that does not pertain simply or directly to the unfolding events. The same sequence of events told by another person to another audience might be presented differently without being any less "true." This is an important point. In contrast with a list of measurements or a description of the outcome of an experiment, there is no self-evident definition of what is relevant or what is irrelevant in a particular narrative. The choice of what to tell and what to omit lies entirely with the narrator and can be modified, at his or her discretion, by the questions of the listener.

This approach gives the physician insight into medicine's four dimensions – physician and patient, physician and self, physician and colleagues, and physicians and society [14]. With narrative competence, physicians can reach and join their patients in illness, recognize their own personal journeys through medicine, acknowledge kinship with and duties toward other health care professionals, and inaugurate consequential discourse with the public about health care. By this approach physicians can integrate their patients as persons with themselves, their colleagues and people in the wider communities and nations to provide renewed opportunities for respectful, empathic, effective, and nourishing medical care.

CONTRASTING MODELS OF MEDICAL CARE

Engels' biopsychosocial model of medicine and the person-centered movement in medicine look broadly at the patient as a person and his or her illness [15]. Narrative provides the means to understand the personal connections between the patient and the physician, the meaning of medical practice for the individual physician, physicians' collective profession of their ideals, and medicine's relationship with the society it serves.

Narrative is concerned with experiences rather than with propositions. Unlike its complement, logic/scientific knowledge, epitomized in evidence-based medicine through which a detached and replaceable observer generates or comprehends replicable and generalizable notices, narrative knowledge of the person leads to local and particular understandings about one situation by one participant or observer. Logic/scientific knowledge attempts to illuminate the universally true by transcending the particular; narrative knowledge attempts to illuminate the universally true by revealing the particular.

The growing narrative sophistication has provided medicine with new and useful ways in which to consider patient–physician relationships, diagnostic reasoning, medical ethics, and professional training. Medicine can, as a result, better understand the experiences of sick people, the journeys of individual physicians, and the duties incurred by physicians toward individual patients and by the profession of medicine toward its wider culture.

INTEGRATING KNOWLEDGE INTO CLINICAL PRACTICE

Sacket and his colleagues found that those who have studied the phenomenon of clinical disagreement, as well as those of us who practice medicine in a clinical setting, know all too well that clinical judgments are usually a far cry from the objective analysis of a set of eminently measurable "facts" [16].

In the language of empiricism such an observation could be interpreted as ascertainment bias [17]. Evidence supports the claim that doctors do not simply assess symptoms and physical signs objectively: they interpret them by integrating the formal diagnostic criteria of the suspected disease (that is, what those diseases are supposed to do in "typical" patients as described in standard textbooks) with the case-specific features of the patient's individual story and their own accumulated professional case expertise. Narrative therefore provides meaning, context, and perspective for a person's predicament. It defines how, why, and in what way he or she is ill [18].

The study of narrative offers a possibility of developing an understanding that cannot be arrived at by any other means. It provides a framework for approaching a person's problems holistically, as well as revealing diagnostic and therapeutic options. Furthermore, narratives of illness provide a medium for the education of both patients and health professionals and may also expand and enrich the research agenda. Indeed, it is thought that anecdotes, or "illness scripts," may be the underlying form in which we accumulate our medical knowledge. Medical students rely on anecdotes of extreme and atypical cases to develop the essential ability to question expectations, interrupt stereotyped thought patterns, and adjust to new developments as a clinical story unfolds [19].

Evidence-based medicine lacks a way of measuring existential qualities such as the inner hurt, despair, hope, grief, and moral pain that frequently accompany, and often indeed constitute, the illnesses from which people suffer. The increasing pursuit during the course of medical training of skills deemed "scientific" and practical, which are readily measurable but inevitably reductionist at the expense of those that are fundamentally linguistic, empathic, and interpretive distorts the clinical method.

It is the core clinical skills of listening, questioning, delineating, organizing explaining, interpreting, and discerning meaning that provide a way of integrating the very different worlds of patients and health professionals. Whether these skills are performed well or badly are likely to have as much influence on the outcome of the illness from the patient's point of view as the more scientific and technical aspects of diagnosis or treatment.

Anecdotal clinical experience may be unrepresentative of the average patient and thus a potentially biased influence on clinical decision making. Evidence-based clinical decision making involves the assessment of the current clinical problem in the light of evidence from the aggregated results of hundreds or thousands of comparable cases in a defined population sample, expressed in the language of probability and risk.

The "truths" established by the empirical observation of populations in randomized trials and cohort studies cannot be mechanistically applied to individuals or episodes of illness where the symptoms and behaviour need to be seen in context.

The generalizable truths gleaned from clinical research trials relate to the samples and, thereby, the study population's story, not the stories of the individual participants. There is a serious danger of erroneously viewing summary statistics as hard realities. Rhi si what has been termed "misplaced concreteness." The dissonance we experience when trying to apply research findings to the clinical encounter often occurs when we abandon the narrative-interpretive paradigm and try to get by on "evidence" alone [20].

MENTAL AND COMORBID CONDITIONS

In the first article of this section of the monograph, Helen Millar [1] illustrates these points in her discussion on person-centered care planning and shared decision making for mental and comorbid conditions with the aim of addressing mental health issues to achieve better compliance with treatment, health and social outcomes and improved quality of life for those living with chronic physical conditions. It is important to recognize the advocacy in the slogan "No health without mental health" [21]. She highlights the developments in the evolving model of person-centered coordinated care in the light of the challenges of the growing epidemic of physical comorbidity in the mentally ill.

She reviews with the key developments supporting proactive and preventative strategies and interventions to tackle comorbidity in this population. Excessive deaths due to comorbidities especially cardiovascular disease continue to contribute to the significant reduction in life expectancy in people with mental health problems. Coordinated collaborative systemwide strategies encompassing shared decision making in prevention and early intervention including lifestyle and pharmacological management are crucial to improve quality of life and life expectancy [22].

We need to help create the conditions for person-centered coordinated care by involving commissioning bodies, patient groups, and practitioners along with community providers. Contemporary models of care for comorbidity emphasize the importance of coordination in the management of physical well-being from the onset of treatment of people with mental health problems in order to ensure better outcomes, improved overall well-being and a longer life expectancy.

ONCOLOGY AND PALLIATIVE CARE

Paul Glare [2] illustrates the importance of shared decision making in oncology and palliative care emphasizing the centrality of the person and the need to understand the risk and benefit in the context of oncological and end-of-life care decisions for each individual [23]. Rapid advances in cancer research, the development of new and more sophisticated approaches to diagnostic testing, and the growth in targeted cancer therapies are transforming the landscape of cancer diagnosis and care. These innovations have contributed to improved outcomes for patients with cancer, but they have also increased the complexity involved in diagnosis and subsequent care decisions. Added to this complexity, focusing on state-of-the-science biomedical treatment may lead to ignoring the psychological and social (psychosocial) problems associated with the illness [24]. Ignoring these issues can compromise the effectiveness of health care and thereby adversely affect the health of cancer patients. Psychological and social problems created or exacerbated by cancer – including depression and other emotional problems – lack of information or skills needed to manage the illness; lack of transportation or other resources; and disruptions in work, school, and family life – cause additional suffering, weaken adherence to prescribed treatments, and threaten patients' return to health [2]. Glare discusses some of the new strategies, which engage appropriate expertise and technologies for treating the disease while ensuring a person-centered approach to caring for cancer patients and their families [25].

SHARED DECISION MAKING FOR OTHER GENERAL CONDITIONS

Appleyard and Snaedal [3] explore the concept of shared decision making in a range of different chronic conditions included within a Cochrane review. The complexities of the decision-making process and the confounding variables create difficulties in obtaining and measuring reproducible outcomes. The beneficial effects of shared decision making including indicators of physical and psychological health status, and people's capability to self-manage their condition when compared to usual care, are greatest when there is more frequent follow-up and continuity of care with the person's personal clinician. "Common ground" is achieved through empathic communication skills with the provision of evidence-based information about options, outcomes, and uncertainties, together with decision support counseling and a systematic approach to recording and implementing patient's preferences.

INTERPROFESSIONAL COLLABORATION

The biomedical, social, psychological mental spiritual needs of a person can only be fulfilled within a team. In the final article of this journal issue, Tesfamicael Ghebrehiwet [4] delineates the key elements that facilitate interprofessional collaboration and identifies the main benefits of and barriers to its development. Interprofessional collaboration in health care occurs when multiple health workers with different professional backgrounds provide person-centered care by working with patients and their families across different settings [26]. It is well accepted that, within each profession, there are varying levels of competence and it is impossible for a single health professional group to provide a continuum of person-centered and cost-effective care [27]. However, the different health professionals can pool their knowledge and expertise to provide person-centered care by working in collaborative practice. For effective collaboration, key barriers must be addressed by the different health professionals. Interprofessional collaboration and communication are largely achieved through interprofessional education during certain periods of their training. Key benefits of interprofessional collaboration and teamwork include fewer medical errors, improved patient outcomes, and better patient safety [28].

REFERENCES

1. Millar H. This issue. Person-Centered Care Planning and Shared Decision-Making for Mental and Comorbid Conditions. International Journal of Person Centered Medicine 8(4): 17–30.
2. Glare P. This issue. Shared Decision Making for Oncological, Chronic Pain and Palliative Care. International Journal of Person Centered Medicine 8(4): 31–40.
3. Appleyard J, Snaedal J. This issue. Shared Decision Making for Other General Conditions. International Journal of Person Centered Medicine 8(4): 41–46.
4. Ghebrehiwet T. This issue. Inter-professional Collaboration for Person-Centered Care. International Journal of Person Centered Medicine 8(4): 47–53.
5. Salzburg Global Seminar. 2011. Salzburg Statement on Shared Decision Making. British Medical Journal 342: d1745.
6. Stacey D, Legare F, Col NF, Bennett CL, Barry MJ, Eden KB, Holmes-Rovner M, Llewellyn-Thomas H, Lyddiatt A, Thomson R, Trevena L, Wu JHC. 2014. Decision Aids for People Facing Health Treatment or Screening Decisions. Cochrane Database of Systematic Reviews 1: CD001431.
7. Coulter A, Entwistle VA, Eccles A, Ryan S, Shepperd S, Perera R. 2015. Personalised Care Planning for Adults with Chronic or Long-Term Health Conditions. Cochrane Database of Systematic Reviews 1: CD010523.
8. Coulter A, Collins A. 2011. Making Shared Decision-Making a Reality, King's Fund, London.
9. Greenhalgh T, Hurwitz B. 1999. Narrative Based Medicine: Why Study Narrative? British Medical Journal 318: 48–50.
10. DeSalvo L. 1999. Writing as a Way of Healing: How Telling Our Stories Transforms Our Lives, Harper, San Francisco, CA.

11. Fox R, Lief H. 1963. Training for "Detached Concern." In: H Lief (Ed). The Psychological Basis of Medical Practice, Harper & Row, New York, pp. 12–35.
12. Jones AH. 1997. Literature and Medicine: Narrative Ethics. Lancet 349: 1243–1246.
15. Engel GL. 1977. The Need for a New Medical Model: A Challenge for Biomedicine. Science196: 129–136.
16. Sackett DL, Rosenberg WMC, Gray JAM, Haynes RB, Richardson WS. 1996. Evidence Based Medicine: What It Is and What It Isn't. British Medical Journal 312: 71.
17. Charon R. 1993. Medical Interpretation Implications of Literary Theory of Narrative for Clinical Work. Journal of Narrative & Life History 3: 79–97.
18. Greenhalgh T, Hurwitz B. 1998. Narrative Based Medicine: Dialogue and Discourse in Clinical Practice, BMJ Books, London.
19. Hurwitz B. 2000. Narrative and the Practice of Medicine. Lancet 356: 2086–2089.
20. Cassell E. 1982. The Nature of Suffering and the Goals of Medicine. New England Journal of Medicine 306: 639–645.
21. Millar H, Abou-Saleh MT. 2011. The World Federation for Mental Health (WFMH) – International Network for Person-Centered Medicine (INPCM) Project: International Journal of Person Centered Medicine 1 (1): 92–97.
22. Adams N. 2012. Finding Common Ground: The Role of Integrative Diagnosis and Treatment Planning as a Pathway to Person-Centered Care. International Journal of Person Centered Medicine 2 (2): 173–178.
23. Weiner JS, Roth J. 2006. Avoiding Iatrogenic Harm to Patient and Family while Discussing Goals of Care Near the End of Life. Journal of Palliative Medicine 9: 451–463.
24. Schnipper LE, Davidson NE, Wollins DS. 2015. A Conceptual Framework to Assess the Value of Cancer Treatment Options. Clinical Oncology 33: 2563–2577.
25. Hoerger M, Epstein RM, Winters PC, Fiscella K, Duberstein PR, Gramling R, Butow PN, Mohile SG, Kaesberg PR, Tang W, Plumb S, Walczak A, Back AL, Tancredi D, Venuti A, Cipri C, Escalera G, Ferro C, Gaudion D, Hoh B, Leatherwood B, Lewis L, Robinson M, Sullivan P, Kravitz RL. 2013. Values and Options in Cancer Care (VOICE): Study Design and Rationale for a Patient-Centered Communication and Decision-Making Intervention for Physicians. BMC Cancer 13: 188.
26. World Health Organization. 2010. Framework for Action on Interprofessional Education & Collaborative Practice. http://www.who.int/hrh/resources/framework_action/en/

27. Ghebrehiwet T. 2015. Inter-Professional Education for Collaborative Practice in Health Care. International Journal of Person Centered Medicine 5: 74–77.
28. Leonard M, Graham S, Bonacum D. 2004. The Human Factor: The Critical Importance of Effective Teamwork and Communication in Providing Safe Care. Quality & Safety in Health Care 13: i85–i90..

PERSON-CENTERED CARE PLANNING AND SHARED DECISION MAKING FOR MENTAL AND COMORBID CONDITIONS

Helen L. Millar, MRCPsych[a] and Ihsan M. Salloum, MD, MPH[b]

ABSTRACT

Developments in person-centered coordinated care are essential given the challenges of the growing epidemic of physical comorbidity in the mentally ill population. Excessive deaths due to comorbidity, especially cardiovascular disease, continue to contribute to the significant reduction in life expectancy in people with mental health problems.

Contemporary and proposed models are now available to provide evidence for a way forward in this field. Practical guidance on implementation using person-centered care planning has now been developed to promote a more collaborative and integrated approach as a solution to the current single disease focused model of care, which is failing this patient group. The WHO perspective supports this strategy with the recent global objectives outlining proactive and preventative strategies and interventions to tackle comorbidity. The emphasis is on a transformation of current systems using evidence-based approaches for more integration to support the delivery of more effective and efficient care for those with mental disorders and other comorbid chronic diseases.

Coordinated, collaborative, system-wide strategies encompass transparent shared decision making in prevention, early intervention, treatment options, lifestyle management and pharmacological rationalization. Hence urgent action is required to help create the conditions to enable the delivery of person-centered coordinated care in health care systems by involving commissioning bodies, clinicians, patient groups along with voluntary and other community providers.

Contemporary models of care for comorbidity emphasize the importance of coordination in the management of physical well-being from the onset of treatment of people with mental health problems in order to ensure better outcomes,

[a] *Consultant Psychiatrist, Queen Margaret Hospital, Scotland, United Kingdom*
[b] *Professor of Psychiatry and Behavioral Sciences, University of Miami Miller School of Medicine, Miami, Florida 33136, United States of America*

improved overall well-being, and a longer life expectancy. Illustratively, no further funds are available to implement this shift in the model of care in the United Kingdom, so redesign and redistribution of current resources will be key to promote this more seamless coordinated system of care to improve the quality of life and life expectancy for this population.

Keywords: person-centered care, shared decision making, mental health, physical health, comorbidity, quality of life, life expectancy, models of care, national health systems, WHO

Correspondence Address: Dr. H. L. Millar, Consultant Psychiatrist, Queen Margaret Hospital, Whitefield Rd, Dunfermline KY12 0SU, Scotland, UK

E-mail: hlmillar1@gmail

INTRODUCTION

The increase in prevalence of comorbidity/multimorbidity continues to be underestimated and hence undertreated resulting in escalating costs to the individual and to society. The consequences for those with mental illness is an excessive burden of disease with an increased risk of cardiovascular disease, cancers, chronic respiratory disorders, and diabetes leading to a reduced life expectancy. Approximately 60% of the excess mortality in the mentally ill is due to general medical conditions [1]. As risk factors for communicable diseases have reduced, the burden of risk factors for NCDs (noncommunicable diseases) has increased. Mental disorders and NCDs share common risk factors and consequences. They are highly interdependent, tend to co-occur, and hence require a more integrated approach [2].

The burden of mental illness and associated comorbidity is expected to increase. By 2030 depression will be ranked number one globally in terms of DALYs (Disability Adjusted Life Years) highlighting the important influence of mental well-being and the need for improved interventions. The WHO has emphasized: "Health is a state of complete physical, mental and social well-being and not simply the lack of disease and infirmity" (WHO 1948). The global mental health plan has highlighted the importance of well-being with the adoption of the slogan "no health without mental health" [3].

Comorbidity is now the norm and not the exception. Hence, there needs to be a recognition that a shift in health care provision is required if we are to address this global phenomenon resulting in an excess burden of disease including premature and preventable causes of mortality in this vulnerable population.

124

The current single disease model fails to provide comprehensive and seamless care. For modern day practitioners, the challenge is how to assess and treat comorbidities. Clinicians currently find themselves caring for individuals in systems, which are fragmented, poorly coordinated, and difficult for both them and patients to navigate through. As a result, there is a failure to deliver key clinical functional outcomes due to a lack of responsiveness to emergency/urgent referrals and rational synchronized long-term management of chronic conditions.

Despite the rhetoric and political support for the integration of health and social services in health care systems in recent years, there still appears to be a marked absence of the practical application of this model. Hence there is still a need to actively transform health care systems to effectively deliver more comprehensive and holistic care to meet the complex overall needs in this population [4].

Along with the integration of the health and social care systems, individual engagement, accountability, and responsibility is key to enhance shared decision making and to improve clinical and functional outcomes. If this is to happen, there needs to be a transformation of the commissioning of health care, a shift in the management and clinical organizational structure, and the delivery of health care to provide the infrastructure for a more responsive and "fit-for-purpose" integrated person-centered model of care.

THE BURDEN AND CHALLENGE OF MENTAL ILLNESS AND COMORBIDITY

Noncommunicable diseases and mental disorders now constitute a large portion of the global burden of disease. The four primary NCDs are cardiovascular disease, chronic respiratory conditions, diabetes, and cancers. Progress has been made to estimate the extent to which mental disorders contribute to the overall disease burden. Over the last 20 years, the evidence demonstrates that there has been a shift of disease burden, measured as Disability Adjusted Life Years (DALYs), from communicable diseases to NCDs, with neuropsychiatric disorders attributing to 28% of the overall disease burden [2].

Mental disorders have been shown to share common features with NCDs in terms of underlying causes and consequences. They also tend to be interdependent and frequently co-occur.

The mechanisms and underlying connections between mental and physical health are complex and suggest a combination of factors: biological, psychosocial, environmental, and behavioral. Hence it is considered that while those with NCDs are at increased risk of mental health problems, there is strong evidence that those with mental health problems such as depression, anxiety, bipolar, or psychotic disorders are more likely to suffer from a range of physical illnesses.

The evidence suggests that the presence of physical health care problems makes diagnosis of a mental illness more difficult. For example, the majority of those suffering depression go undetected and untreated in those with physical health problems. Also, there is evidence to suggest that access to physical health checks for those with mental disorders is more limited for a wide variety of reasons [5].

Research to date demonstrates that those suffering from long-term NCDs are two to three times more likely to suffer from mental health problems. Much of the evidence points to affective disorders such as depression and anxiety although comorbidities are also common in bipolar disorder, schizophrenia, dementia, cognitive decline, and other conditions. Overall the evidence suggests that at least 30% of those with long-term conditions have a mental health problem [6, 7].

NCDs show common risk factors that are modifiable such as poor diet, lack of exercise, harmful use of alcohol, and use of tobacco. Excessive smoking, poor diet, obesity, misuse of substances, and a sedentary lifestyle are more common in those with mental illness than in the general population.

It is now evidenced that mental health problems such as depression when associated with physical health conditions namely asthma, diabetes, or congestive cardiac problems dramatically increase the medical costs of care. Much of the costings quoted in the literature gathered from the US health care system demonstrate an increase by 33% to 169% across a range of physical health conditions when associated with depression and anxiety. A study based on US insurance claims showed that depression increased costs by between 50% and 190% when associated with conditions such as asthma, congestive heart failure, and diabetes [8].

Depression studies have shown that this mental health problem can impact on the individual's ability to cope and manage long-term conditions such as diabetes leading to worsened functional outcomes, disability, more complications, and worse prognosis. Poor pharmacotherapy compliance and dietary control can result from poor motivation in managing a healthy lifestyle [9, 10].

In addition those with mental health comorbidity are less likely to work, productivity when working is reduced and high levels of absenteeism are reported.

International research studies demonstrate that the bulk of excess costs are associated with the most complex patients with long-term conditions who suffer the most severe illnesses or who have multiple comorbidities [6].

People with mental health problems have the additional burden of potential adverse effects caused by long-term prescribed psychotropic medication. The more commonly used second generation of antipsychotics are a heterogeneous group of drug with varying degrees of cardiometabolic risks including weight gain, dyslipidaemia, and an increased potential for diabetes [11]. This cluster of cardiometabolic risk factors have been termed "metabolic syndrome" in an attempt to assist clinicians to target screening of high-risk individuals. There has been increasing controversy over this term. Overall it has been considered useful in clinical settings to estimate the prevalence of this problem in groupings such as schizophrenia and bipolar disorder, which has been estimated in international surveys at 42% and 22–30%, respectively [1].

The management of multimorbidity for the physician can, at times, be overwhelming given the complexity in pharmacotherapy required for treatment of the comorbid physical and mental disorders resulting in, at times, high levels of polypharmacy. The management of such individuals requires ongoing close monitoring of medications, regular rationalization of drugs to ensure that the risk benefit ratio is reviewed and that the most effective combinations are utilized with the optimum benefit and minimum adverse effects.

For the individual it can be challenging to recall when to take medications prescribed and hence adhere to the polypharmacy regime despite their best efforts. In addition it can be difficult to coordinate and attend the numerous specialist appointments and multiple investigations at different health care centers. At times tests can be double booked and repeated unnecessarily by different specialists due to the lack of communication and joint up health care records. Care can seem uncoordinated for these individuals leading to a sense of confusion and lack of clarity of priorities in functional outcomes and treatment goals. At times the individual can receive what seems to be conflicting advice from different specialists depending on their own treatment goals and priorities and their level of expertise.

Hence the management of comorbidity with mental illness is challenging from both the clinicians' and the patient's perspective. Guidelines have focused on a single disease model of care, but there appears to be an increasing awareness of the need to improve the life of those with multimorbidity by reducing treatment burden and unplanned care. The aim is now directed at taking into account multimorbidity, what approach would most likely benefit the individual, how they can be identified, and what the care will involve. Hence to improve the overall quality of life, shared decision making is crucial in terms of the clinician and patient jointly reviewing treatment options, weighing up health priorities, and setting clear lifestyle goals.

GLOBAL PLAN FOR THE DELIVERY OF PERSON-CENTERED CARE FOR COMORBIDITY INCLUDING MENTAL ILLNESS

The WHO highlighted the challenge of the world's most common diseases in the global action plan (2013–2020). With more than 14 million people between 30 and 70 years of age dying from NCDs every year and more than 85% living in developing countries.

The strategy calls for strengthened leadership and national capacity to drive the process, promote high-quality research, track trends, and monitor the program's success. The main message is prevention and control of NCDs, which has among its goals a 25% relative reduction in premature mortality due to NCDs by 2025 (the so-called 25 x 25 goal) through targeting of seven risk factors namely tobacco use, harmful use of alcohol, physical inactivity, sodium intake, raised blood pressure, obesity, and diabetes [12].

This plan was followed up by the WHO's comprehensive plan for an integrated approach to mental disorders and NCDs (WHO (2014) as a response to the fundamental connection between mental disorders and NCDs and the implications in terms of health care systems. The emphasis is on a transformation of the delivery of health care from the single disease model to an integrated collaborative approach, which is effective and efficient to manage mental disorders and other chronic conditions. The challenge was clearly outlined as a transformation of health care systems not simply scaling up current structures. The point of the integration is to fundamentally provide benefits to both patients and the health system by providing increased accessibility, reduce fragmentation to better meet the needs of this population [5].

The principles and actions required are clarified from a public health approach along with a shift in systems, government engagement, and collaboration. The overarching approach must start in the prenatal period and continue through the life course from infancy, adolescence through to adulthood with the promotion of healthy lifestyle behaviors and coordinated and continuous care. There must be governance in the system to promote accurate data collection, HR support with financial rationalization, and prioritization. Clinicians and service users must be involved in fundamental decisions and there must be transparency and collaboration across sectors to create opportunities for integrated care and support.

Since it is now established that there are such strong links between mental disorders and NCDs, it is clear that the only feasible way to prevent and effectively manage comorbidity is though a seamless integrated person-centered model of care. This care model must include targeting those with the long-term conditions and comorbid mental health problems to enable self-referral and self-management and encourage joint accountability and responsibility.

The International College of Person Centered Care Medicine's 2014 Geneva Declaration on Person- and People-Centered Integrated Health Care for All [13] provided six key domains for this:

• Person- and People-Centered Integrated Health Care (PPCIC) integrate the relationship between the people seeking and those delivering care so that it is health care:

- Of the person, i.e., address the whole person
- For the person, i.e., to promote the person's health and well-being fulfillment
- By the person, i.e., including the person of the health professional
- With the person, i.e., in respectful and empowering collaboration with the person presenting for care
- PPCIC is planned and delivered within the social network of each person
- PPCIC ensures coordination of health care over their life time
- PPCIC promotes vertical integration within the health care sector by planning and coordinating care among primary care givers and specialists
- PPCIC promotes horizontal integration across multiple sectors of society
- PPCIC promotes the shared vision of well-being for all people

CURRENT MODELS FOR PERSON-CENTERED PLANNING AND SHARED DECISION MAKING

Health care systems are actively responding to the move toward integration and a more person-centered approach, but given the current pressures, efforts tend to be inconsistent and patchy. The United Kingdom has recognized that in order to progress further there needs to be a culture shift involving the whole system supported by the entire organization, i.e., individual practitioners, multidisciplinary teams, provider organizations, and commissioners. Realistic evaluation of the whole system must address service redesign, implementation, education, and proper evaluation and research.

The recent Lancet Commission article emphasizes the need for protecting physical health in people with mental illness and views it as an international priority. The article highlights the large disparities that still exist in the physical health of those with mental illness despite awareness in the field and the need for better integration of services for mental and physical health care. Strategies are clearly outlined including; further global recognition of primary prevention through recognition of shared risk factors, implementation of a culture shift through development of local, national, and international policies, further research in the field to provide more robust evidence focusing on prevention/ screening of comorbidities, early intervention, and the delivery of practical lifestyle interventions along with monitoring of long-term side effects of psychotropic medication [14].

A contemporary reality-based example of a person-centered approach is P3C (person-centered coordinated care). This framework was developed to accelerate the spread and wider implementation of person-centered care in a practical way in the United Kingdom [15].

P3C was developed by the Plymouth University Pennisula Group, which was originally set up to address the management of long-term conditions and those at the end of life to provide a portfolio of intelligence on the use of metrics for person-centered coordinated care [16].

Practical guidance and templates have now been developed by this research group to assist with implementation of person-centered coordinated care with essential feedback loops to measure success. The program is seen as a collaborative effort looking at recognition of problems in practice and generating whole system improvements through evaluation of specific initiatives with built-in reviews and specific clinically based research projects [17].

The data collection included (1) a rapid evidence scan to synthesis evidence for the use of Patient Reported Measures (PRMs) to improve the quality of care for the patient group, (2) an exploration of the use of PRMs from a collection of stories, (3) views from stakeholder groups to explore the use of PRMs, (4) a survey to capture experiences of commissioners, (5) production of an on line compendium of measurements to assess P3C, and (6) a guide to support commissioners to deliver P3C.

Evidence from a number of systematic reviews suggests that PRMs can improve the quality of care in a number of ways: Firstly, they have been used as a tool to evaluate interventions in clinical trials. Secondly, PRMs can act as essential feedback to clinicians and patients to support decision making for diagnostic processing, prioritizing treatment goals, and improving overall decision making through the phases of the patient's journey. Thirdly, health care providers can use the PRMs for benchmarking, audits, quality improvement, and commissioning.

PRMs can be helpfully used in a multidirectional manner and act as system's tools to aggregate data for quality improvement for clinicians. This aggregated data can then be shared with the public to promote quality improvement, influence consumer choice and improve public accountability. PRMs are being designed to evaluate a variety of health care outcomes and experiences from the patient perspective as well as from the family and carers' view point. Person-centered care patient reported measures' (PCC-PRMs) domains such as communication, self–management, and patient activation have been utilized. Other measures can include quality of life and health-related quality of life.

The evaluation framework includes feedback from patients, teams, and the organization to gain a multiperspective and multilevel measure of change with specified measures of success.

The practice of PCC is still being established, evidenced, and documented. The essence of PCC involves active listening, agreeing, and formulating a plan based on shared decision making and preferences of the patient working in partnership and documenting this in a cocreated care plan. The plan requires coordination with other professionals.

130

The move toward a more "healthy relationship" with the patient is crucial in our current health care environment. The idea being that the practice of P3C can provide a mechanism for experiential learning for both the practitioner and the patient and allow for new ways for reflecting thinking and working.

A recent updated study in this field by Wheat et al. (2018) was completed to explore how professionals use PRMs to enhance P3C and measure whether person-centered coordinated care (P3C) was actually being delivered [18].

As discussed, patient reported measures (PRMs) have been used to provide a measurement of patients' experiences of P3C. In the past they have been used to assess whether interventions are delivering P3C. There has been an increased interest in their potential use in helping to improve practitioner–patient communication. However, to date, there is limited research available on how P3C can be implemented in practice.

This study explored how professionals use PRMs to enhance P3C. Themes were mapped onto components of P3C care that fell under five established domains of P3C (Information and Communication, My Goals/Outcomes, Decision Making, Care Planning, and Transitions) to explore whether and how individual components of P3C were being improved through PRMs. Barriers and facilitators that affected the delivery and the results of the PRMs were also identified. Results: Three P3C domains (Information and Communication, My Goals/Outcomes, and Care Planning) were mapped frequently onto themes generated by the participants' interviews about PRM use. However, the domain "Decision Making" was only mapped onto one theme and "Transitions" was not mapped at all. Participant reports suggested that PRM use by practitioners enhanced patients' ability to self-manage, communicate, engage, and reflect during consultations.

The study confirmed that the barriers to PRM use were related to a lack of a "whole service" approach to implementation. The study concluded that practitioners can use both PROMs and PREMs (patient-reported outcome measures and patient-reported experience measures) to improve different aspects of patient care. By sharing experiences professionals can benefit from each other's learning and work together to extend the potential value that PRMs can offer to P3C delivery.

Within the United Kingdom, this model has been utilized in the roll out of a government initiative described as the "House of Care," which provides a framework for personalized care and support planning encouraging care professionals to work with those with long-term conditions including both physical and mental health problems. The personalized care and support planning is a process in which the person with a long-term condition is active in the care through a continuous process with monitoring of progress. The conditions being treated are those that cannot be cured but are managed or improved to ensure the best quality of life for the individual while living and that they die as humanely as possible. The essential ingredient in this form of personalized care and support planning is that the person with the long-term condition is an equal and active partner in the process, which should take place effectively with the process being recorded in the personalized support plan [19].

This method of long-term care can help to utilize finite resources more appropriately. People who are engaged in their health care are more likely to receive care and treatment that is appropriate to them: regular screening, healthy lifestyle behavior, successful self-management, and by anticipating and making explicit provision for crises and emergencies can help reduce the need for emergency care and services.

The Francis report in the United Kingdom brought into sharp focus the lack of empathy and compassion in the NHS and the need to refocus on the individual's needs and their families and be responsive to the individual's strengths and resources. Person-centered care is a way of achieving such goals for individuals with complex health and social needs and addressing the demands and inefficiencies within the current system. It is also being envisaged as an answer to the present economic shortfalls and improve efficiency. This vision is based on the perception that by seeing the individual as a whole person this will help professionals and services organize care more efficiently and enhance coordination of care [20].

NICE guidance supports this model for the management of "Multimorbidity" by focusing on optimizing care for adults with multiple long-term conditions by reducing treatment burden and unplanned care. It aims at improving quality of life by promoting shared decision making based on the person's health priorities, lifestyle, and goals. The guideline highlights who is likely to benefit from this approach taking into account multimorbidity, how they are identified, and what the care involves [21].

The Person-Centered Care Index (PCI), developed by the International College of Person Centered Medicine, provides a suitable metric to measuring person- and people-centeredness of care, "i.e., addressing the whole person." The PCI systematically assesses the degree to which care is delivered according to the tenant of person-centered medicine. Key concepts underlying person-centered medicine measured by the PCI include the following eight domains: (1) Ethical Commitment, (2) Cultural Sensitivity, (3) Holistic scope, (4) Relational Focus, (5) Individualized Care, (6) Common Ground for Collaborative Diagnosis and Care, (7) People-centered Systems of Care, and (8) Person-centered Education and Research. These domains are assessed through 33 subitems, each measured on a 4-point scale. The PCI has high Cronbach internal consistency and scale unidimensionality as well as high inter-rater reliability and substantial content validity [22]. The PCI is being used internationally, particularly in Latin America, to evaluate person-centeredness in health services [23].

CONCLUSIONS

Person-centered medicine is an emerging field that emphasizes the whole person, the totality of their health status including ill health as well as positive aspects of health and well-being, including the contributors to health (ill health and well-being) in a biopsychosocial framework. It empowers the therapeutic relationship and views the health care provider and the person presenting for care to be in a partnership with common goals. Without shared responsibility and shared decision making, this model of delivering care is not feasible.

Although the concept of person-centered care has been well established, further education and training is required to shift the current thinking on how care is delivered.

It is clear that our current uncoordinated health and social system of care is failing patients who present with complex long-term conditions. The original chronic conditions model of care proposed a comprehensive system based on a bio-psycho-social model, which is as relevant now as it was when originally released [24].

If we are to move toward a truly person-centered approach to care and work in a more integrated and seamless collaborative way, practical reality-tested models and templates are now available. If the system is to refocus from the single disease model to the whole person model, health systems have to be engaged in moving forward. The person-centered coordinated care model – P3C in the United Kingdom embraces person-centered care and acts as a platform to facilitate the necessary framework to implement this coherent approach with inbuilt monitoring/auditing of progress, supporting practical developments, and promoting healthy communication. The PCI provides a broad internationally suitable and practical systematic assessment of person-centeredness in care. It incorporates shared decision making and agreed treatment goals as does the United Kingdom's person-centered co-ordinated model to optimize outcomes for those with complex long-term conditions.

Hence, an optimistic and constructive approach is evolving, utilizing evidence-based research to date, implementing national/international policies and guidelines and delivering practical models that have been developed to improve person-centered care. It is only by promoting this culture shift to a more collaborative holistic model of care that we can improve outcomes for people with mental illness and comorbid conditions.

ACKNOWLEDGMENTS AND DISCLOSURES

The authors do not report any conflicts of interest concerning this paper.

REFERENCES

1. Marc DE Hert, Christoph U Correll, Julio Bobes, Marcelo Cetkovich-Bakmas, Dan Cohen, Itsuo Asai, Johan Detraux, Shiv Gautam, Hans-Jurgen Möller, David M Ndetei, John W Newcomer, Richard Uwakwe, Stefan Leucht 2011. Physical Illness in Patients with Severe Mental Disorders. World Psychiatry 10: 52–77.
2. Ngo VK, Rubenstein A, Ganju V, Kanellis P, Loza N, Rabadan C, Daar AS. Grand Challenges: Integrating Mental Health Care into the Non-communicable Disease Agenda 2013. PLOS Med 10(5): e 1001443, doi: 10,1371/ journal. pmed.1001443
3. Prince M, Patel V, Shekhar S, Maj M, Maselko J, Philips MR, Rahman A, Maselko J. 2007. No Health without Mental Health. Lancet 370: 859–877.
4. World Health Organization. 2015. Global Strategy on People Centred and Integrated Health Services, World Health Organization.
5. World Health Organization and Calouste Gulbenkian Foundation. 2014. Integrating the Response to Mental Disorders and Other Chronic Diseases in Health Care Systems, World Health Organization, Geneva.
6. Naylor C, Parsonage M, McDaid D, Knapp M, Fossey M, Galea A. 2012. Long-Term Conditions and Mental Health: The Cost of Co-morbidities, The King's Fund for Mental Health, London.
7. Cimpean D, Drake RE. 2011. Treating Co-morbid Medical Conditions and Anxiety/Depression. Epidemiology and Psychiatric Service 20: 141–150.
8. Welch CA, Czerwinski D, Ghimire B, Bertsimas D. 2009. Depression and Costs of Health Care. Pscyhosomatics 50: 392–401.
9. Hutter N, A Schnurr A, H Baumeister H. 2010. Healthcare Costs in Patients with Diabetes Mellitus and Co-morbid Mental Disorders: A Systematic Review. Diabetologia 53: 2470–2479.
10. Moussavi S, Chatterji S, Verdes E, Tandon A, Patel V, Ustun B 2007. Depression, Chronic Diseases and Decrements in Health: Results from the World Health Surveys. Lancet 370: 851–858.
11. Sinha A, Shariq A, Said K, Sharma A, Jeffrey Newport D, Salloum IM. 2018. Medical Comorbidities in Bipolar Disorder. Current Psychiatry Reports 20(5): 36.
12. World Health Organization. 2013. World Health Action Plan 2013–2020: Global Action Plan for the Prevention and Control of NCDs 2013–2020, World Health Organization, Geneva.

13. International College of Person Centered Medicine. 2014. The 2104 Geneva Declaration on Person centered and People centered Integrated Health Care for All. International Journal of Person Centered Medicine 4: 66–68.
14. Firth J, Siddiqi N, Koyanagi A, Siskind D, Rosenbaum S, Galletly C, Allan S, Caneo C, Carney R, Carvalho A F, Chatterton M L, Correll C U, Curtis J, Gaughran F, Heald A, Hoare E, Jackson S E, Kisely S, Lovell K, Maj M, McGorry P D, Mihalopoulos C, Myles H, O'Donoghue B, Pillinger T, Sarris J, Schuch F B, Shiers D, Smith L, Solmi M, Suetani S, Taylor J, Teasdale S B, Thornicroft G, Torous J, Usherwood T, Vancampfort D, Veronese N, Ward P B, Yung A, Killackey E, Stubbs B 2019. The Lancet Psychiatry Commission: A Blue Pront for Protecting Physical Health in People with Mental Illness. The Lancet Psychiatry 6: 675–712.
15. Horrell J, Lloyd H, Sugavanam T, Close J, Byng R. 2017. Creating and Facilitating Change for Person-Centered Co-ordinated Care (P3C): The development of the Organisational Change Tool (P3C-OCT). Health Expectations 21: 448–456.
16. Lloyd H, Pearson M, Sheaff R, Asthana S, Wheat H, Thava Priya Sugavanam 5, Nicky Britten N, Valderas J, Bainbridge M, Witts L, Westlake D, Jane Horrell J, Byng R. 2017. Collaborative Action for Person-Centered Co-ordinated Care (P3C): An Approach to Support the Development of a Comprehensive System-wide Solution to Fragmented Care. Health Research Policy and systems 15: 98.
17. P3C Commissioners Guide. 2017. Person Centred Coordinated Care Programme, South West Peninsula CLAHRC. Plymouth University Peninsula Schools of Medicine and Dentistry Room: http://clahrc-peninsula.nihr.ac.uk/research/person-centred-coordinated-care-p3c; https://www.plymouth.ac.uk/research/primarycare/person-centred-coordinated-care
18. Wheat H, Horrell J, Valderas J M, J Close J, Fosh B, Lloyd H. 2018. Can Practitioners Use Patient Reported Measures to Enhance Person Centred Coordinated Care in Practice? A Qualitative Study. Health and Quality of Life Outcomes 16: 223.
19. NHS. 2016. NHS England Personalised care and support planning handbook. The journey to person centered care. Person Centred Care/Coalition for Collaborative Care/Medical Directorate, NHS, London.
20. Report of the Mid Staffordshire NHS Foundation Trust; Public Inquiry Feb 2013.
21. NICE Multimorbidity https://www.nice.org.uk/guidance/ng56
22. Mezzich JE, Kirisci L, Salloum IM, Trivedi JK, Kar SK, Adams N, Wallcraft J. 2016. Systematic Conceptualization of Person Centered Medicine and Development and Validation of a Person-centered Care Index. International Journal of Person Centered Medicine 6 (4): 219–247.

23. Perales A, Kirisci L, Mezzich JE, Sánchez E, Barahona L, Zavala S, Amorín E. 2018. Comparative Study of Prototype Hospitals in Lima with the Person-Centered Care Index Rated by Health Professionals. International Journal of Person Centered Medicine 8: 47–65.
24. Wagner EH. 1998. Chronic Disease Management: What Will It Take to Improve Care for Chronic Illness? Effective Clinical Practice 1 (1): 2–4.

SHARED DECISION MAKING IN ONCOLOGY AND PALLIATIVE CARE

Paul Glare, MBBS, FRACP, FAChPM RACP, FFPMANZCA[a]

ABSTRACT

Background: Cancer raises many questions for people afflicted by it. Do I want to have genetic testing? Will I comply with screening recommendations? If I am diagnosed with it, where will I have treatment? What treatment modalities will I have? Will I go on a clinical trial? Am I willing to bankrupt my family in the process of pursuing treatment? Will I write an advance care plan? Will I accept hospice if I have run out of available treatment options? Most of these questions have more than one correct answer, and the evidence for the superiority of one option over another is either not available or does not allow differentiation. Often the best choice between two or more valid approaches depends on how individuals value their respective risks and benefits; "preference-based medicine" may be more important than "evidence-based medicine." There are various models for eliciting preferences, but applying them can raise a number of challenges.

Objectives: To present the concepts, the value, the strategies, the quandaries, and the potential pitfalls of Shared Decision Making in Oncology and Palliative Care.

Method: Narrative review.

Results: Some challenges to practicing preference-based medicine in oncology and palliative care include: some patients don't want to participate in shared decision making (SDM); the whole situation needs to be addressed, not just part of it; but are some topics out of bounds? Cognitive biases apply as much in SDM as any other human decision making, affecting the choice; how numerically equivalent data are framed can also affect the outcome; conducting SDM is also important at the end of life.

Conclusions: By being aware of the potential pitfalls with SDM, clinicians are more able to facilitate the discussion so that the patients' choices truly reflect their informed preferences, at a time when stakes and emotions are high.

―――――――――――――――――

[a] *Specialist Physician in Pain Medicine and Palliative Care*
Professor, Sydney Medical School
Head of Discipline Pain Medicine, Sydney Medical Program
Director, Pain Management Research Institute, Faculty of Medicine & Health
University of Sydney, NSW, Australia

Correspondence Address: Postal address: Prof. Paul Glare, Pain Management Research Centre, Level 2, Douglas Building, Royal North Shore Hospital, Reserve Rd., St Leonards NSW 2065, Australia

E-mail address: paul.glare@sydney.edu.au

Keywords: shared decision making, oncology, palliative care, person-centered medicine, treatment planning, preference-based medicine, evidence-based medicine, choices/options/decision talk prospect theory

INTRODUCTION

Cancer raises many questions for people afflicted by it. Do I want to have genetic testing? Will I comply with screening recommendations? If I am diagnosed with it, where will I have treatment? What treatment modalities will I have? Will I go on a clinical trial? Am I willing to bankrupt my family in the process of pursuing treatment? Will I write an advance care plan? Will I accept hospice if I have run out of available treatment options?

Most of these questions have more than one correct answer, and the evidence for the superiority of one option over another is either not available or does not allow differentiation. In some situations (e.g., patient has a specific tumor mutation, or is septic and hypotensive from febrile neutropenia), the patient may be content with having an oncologist making evidence-based decisions on their behalf, e.g., which biological agent to choose, whether to admit to hospital. But often the best choice between two or more valid approaches depends on how individuals value their respective risks and benefits [1], and "preference-based medicine" is more important than evidence-based medicine [2].

Shared decision making (SDM) is the result of practicing preference-based medicine. SDM requires the person with the illness to think about the available screening, treatment, or management options and the likely benefits and harms of each so that they can communicate their preferences and help select the best course of action for them. SDM requires building a good relationship in the clinical encounter so that information is shared and patients are supported to deliberate and express their preferences and views during the decision-making process. The model has three steps: (1) introducing choice, (2) describing options, often by integrating the use of patient decision support, and (3) helping patients explore preferences and make decisions. This model rests on supporting a process of deliberation, and on understanding that decisions should be influenced by exploring and respecting "what matters most" to patients as individuals, and that this exploration in turn depends on them developing informed preferences. To facilitate this approach, a practical three-step model has been developed, built around the three conversations that are need for SDM: Choice Talk, Option Talk, and Decision Talk [3].

SHARED DECISION MAKING IN ONCOLOGY

One of the most well-publicized oncology decisions was that made by Angelina Jolie to have a prophylactic mastectomy and to have made her own decision. We can only speculate how Ms. Jolie made her decision. But the report in Time Magazine in 2013 [4] gives some insight into how the three-step choice/options/ decision-talk model might have helped her and her oncologist make the decision that fit best with her disease and her preferences (see Box 1).

While using a model like Choices/Options/Decision Talk can be seen to help SDM, physicians are likely to face a number of challenges when practicing SDM

Box 1. How the Choice/Options/Talk Model can facilitate shared decision making in oncology

- **CHOICE TALK:** Yes, Ms. Jolie, the choices are prophylactic surgery or regular screening. There are no effective drug treatments.
- **OPTIONS TALK:** There is a 90% chance you will get breast cancer or ovarian cancer.
    - Extensive surgery will drastically reduce the risk but not eliminate it.
    - If found early with screening, 5-year survival after breast cancer treatment is almost 100%, and >90% for ovarian cancer.
    - Screening is good for breast cancer but not simple for ovarian cancer.
    - Screening has no side effects. Surgery side effects include body image and pain.
- **DECISION TALK:** If your goal is a sense of relief by minimizing your cancer risk by doing whatever it takes then you may want to choose prophylactic surgery.
    - If you wish to avoid surgery, choose screening even though the risks are slightly higher.
    - Other factors like your celebrity status and your children may be relevant.

in day-to-day practice. The aim of this paper is to consider some of them so that clinicians are aware of them and how to manage them.

1. Not every patient is interested in SDM

Aside from emergent situations that preclude SDM, as mentioned previously, factors like age, gender, marital status, culture (and acculturation), religion, education, and health literacy may influence an individual's preferred style of decision making. The stage of the illness may also be relevant. For example, a survey of 78 Canadian patients with advanced cancer indicated that only two-thirds wanted to participate in SDM [5]. However, the patients' physicians underestimated this proportion, correctly predicting patient preference in less than 50% cases. Neither age nor gender was predictive of decision-making preference in this study. Mood could also be relevant: a depressed or anxious patient may have difficulty with SDM.

2. The whole situation needs to be discussed, not just some aspects of it

The consequences of discussing an oversimplified version of a decision have been analyzed for a geriatric oncology case [6]. The case describes an elderly patient with lung cancer that has progressed despite conventional chemotherapy. He reports pain, short of breath on exertion, and anorexia, but is still ambulant. The oncologist recommends a trial of immunotherapy. But the internist who is present recommends palliative care/hospice. During the Options Talk, the oncologist states that 20–40% patients respond to immunotherapy with a median survival of 15 months; without treatment, the median survival is only 8 months. The internist recommends palliative care and hospice because it will ensure 8 months of good quality time. The family chose chemotherapy.

In analyzing the decision, the authors refer to Prospect Theory [6]. Prospect Theory states that when people face overwhelmingly complex decisions, they tend to compensate by taking a number of mental short cuts, which can be missteps:

- they focus on one aspect, at the cost of oversimplifying the situation;
- they frame the choices for that one aspect as gains or losses;
- being generally loss averse, they are more willing to take risks (to avoid the pain of losses), and only pursue gains if they are certainties;
- they tend to focus on the short-term outcomes only.

In this case, the oncologist and family were seen to be focusing on survival; they were ignoring other issues, like quality of life, place of care, cost of care, mode of death. The oncologist and family were focused on the loss of 7 months of life without immunotherapy and were willing to take that risk even though the chance of achieving it was low. The authors proposed that the family may not have chosen more treatment if they were encouraged to think about the whole situation (side effects of treatment, need for frequent appointments and potential hospitalization, quality of life, cost of care), not just the oversimplified version; and to be aware of other persuasive forces that influence choice.

3. But is anything out of bounds in the discussion?

Shared decision making (SDM) encourages patients to think about all the available screening, treatment, or management options and the likely benefits and harms of each so that they can communicate their preferences and help select the best course of action for them. But does the physician have a duty to present every single option, even if they think it is inappropriate? For example are they obliged to discuss prognosis? Many physicians avoid prognosticating as they are untrained in how to do it, don't want to "play God" and fear how they will be judged if they are inaccurate [7]. Or cost? Patients may feel uncomfortable discussing costs of their treatment options with physicians, while some physicians feel ill prepared to undertake a dialogue involving costs [8].

4. Other cognitive biases also affect choice

In addition to oversimplification of complex choices, people use various other "mental rules of thumb," or heuristics, facilitate decision making in the face of uncertainty. Like any short cut, heuristics are often effective but are prone to error. The result is biased thinking and making suboptimal choices.

The list of cognitive biases is long. Some of the common ones that could be problematic in medical decision making include:

- "Optimism" bias: believing that I will be the 1-in-10 that responds to this Phase I clinical trial agent
- "Availability" bias: tendency to recall what's in front of one's mind, e.g., latest cancer miracle or celebrity case reported in the news
- "Confirmation" bias: tendency to recall cases that support one's opinion, while ignoring those that don't

5. Do people really act autonomously when making a shared decision?

Even when we choose shared decision making, people tend to act in certain ways that could prevent them fully participating in the process:

- We want to be liked, including by our physician
- We want to be consistent in our decisions
- We want to be good, as we expect generosity to be reciprocated
- We believe what we are told
- We are obedient to authority

6. How the data are framed can affect the choice?

Making preference-based decisions involves the person with the disease operating in uncertainty and weighing up risks of multiple options, a process they may not be familiar with. Decision aids and other tools are available to support them but even then, it is well known that people react differently to how numbers depending on how they are framed.

A classic example is documented in an older study, published in the NEJM nearly half a century ago, on people's preferences for two lung cancer treatments, A or B [9]. In the scenario, Treatment A causes some deaths at the time of treatment but has a better long-term outcome. Treatment B causes no deaths at the time of treatment but has a worse long-term outcome. The proportions and outcomes were framed in various ways that were numerically identical (i.e., 10% succeed vs. 90% fail). The study found that preferences flipped from A to B depending on how the data were presented. Short-term outcome was presented as 10% chance of dying after Treatment A (in which case prefer B) to 90% chance of surviving after Treatment A (prefer A). Long-term outcome was described as survival (prefer A) vs. cumulative mortality (prefer B). Treatment A was also preferred when it was revealed to be surgery and Treatment B was revealed to be radiation therapy.

7. How the data are presented also matters [9]?

Other studies have shown that people's preferences change when equivalent numerical data are presented in different ways [10]. Some examples include:

- A fraction vs. a percentage (e.g., one-in-five vs. 20%)
- A percentage (e.g., 20%) vs. a category (e.g., common, possible, unlikely)
- Aggregated results (median 15 months) vs. disaggregated results (6 months: 80%, 1 year: 60%; 2 years 30%; 5 years 10%)
- Average case vs. Best case vs. worse case

- Reduction of risk from 100% to 80% vs. reduction from 20% to 0%.
- Relative risk reduction vs. absolute risk reduction (reduction from 96% to 94% framed as a 33% relative risk reduction vs. a 2% absolute risk reduction)

SPECIFIC CHALLENGES TO SHARED DECISION MAKING IN PALLIATIVE CARE AND AT THE END OF LIFE

All of the challenges to shared decision making that occur earlier in the cancer journey can occur at the end of life. As with the geriatric oncology case above, patients/families can be reluctant to transition from cancer treatment to palliative care/hospice. And in the terminal stages they may demand "everything" be done to prolong life even when the patient has entered the terminal phase.

1. Patient/family dislikes the option that physician is recommending as best in the circumstances

Patients and their family may dislike some recommendations included in the Choice/Option Talk, such as hospice enrolment, even if that option best meets their needs at this stage of the illness. An approach that may be effective in this situation is to apply the principles of Regulatory Focus theory [11]. The ancient Greeks identified that people are motivated to seek pleasure and avoid pain. More recently, the principle of regulatory focus predicts that how people seek pleasure/ avoid pain is determined by whether they tend to have more of a "promotion" focus (motivated by accomplishments and aspirations) or a predominantly "prevention" focus (motivated by safety and responsibilities) [11]. Moreover, Prospect Theory shows that we are often motivated to avoid pain (losses) than seek pleasure (gains) [6]. In a health care setting, a promotion focus person would be motivated to quit smoking to get fitter, while a prevention focus person would be motivated to quit to avoid dying. The regulatory focus theory is extended by considering whether messages fit with a person's focus or not. "Smoking ages your skin" fits a promotion focus and motivates such a person to quit; "don't let your children inhale your smoke" fits a prevention focus and motivates such a person more than it motivates a promotion focus person. In fact statements that don't fit the persons focus ("non-fit statements") tend to be demotivating [12].

Some research has shown that the demotivating effect of regulatory non-fit statements can be used to de-intensify negative attitudes to disliked recommendations, such as the transition from oncology treatment to hospice. Regulatory non-fit de-intensifies participants' initial attitudes by making them less confident in their initial judgments and motivating them to think more thoroughly about the arguments presented. Furthermore, consistent with previous research on regulatory fit, the mechanism of regulatory non-fit differs as a function of participants' cognitive involvement in the evaluation of the hospice option [13]. Because a person's motivational focus can be primed, e.g., by getting them to think about times when they were operating in promotion mode or prevention mode, clinicians don't need to determine a dissatisfied patient's regulatory focus first before presenting a non-fit statement about more treatment or hospice [14].

2. The patient and family want "everything" done to prolong life in a dying patient

In terms of shared decision making for the patient/family who wants "everything," a panel of communication experts from US palliative care have provided a useful two-step framework (see Box 2) to assist clinicians who are committed to SDM to resolve such impasses [15]. The first step involves clarifying what "everything" means, in terms of where the patient/family lie on the quality of life risk-benefit continuum. Palliative sedation lies at one end and coding multiple times in ICU at the other. Unless the patient/family lie at the extreme end of high risk/low benefit, a compromise may well be achieved just by clarifying the limits to "everything."

If a compromise can't be reached, then the second step utilizes good communication skills to explore why the patient/family feel so strongly. Using a biopsychosocial framework, areas to explore include a knowledge deficit about the disease stage and the treatment options; affective problems such as depression or anxiety; psychosocial stressors such as complex family dynamics or young children; or a spiritual issue such as fundamentalist religious beliefs.

Exploring these issues may identify modifiable factors that allow an agreement

Box 2. An approach to achieving a consensus with a patient/family who want overly aggressive treatment at end of life

Task	Communication issues
1. Clarify attitude to risks vs. benefits	How far willing to go to achieve outcome?
2. Explore potential issues	
• Cognitive	Clarify diagnosis, treatment options, prognosis
• Affective	Evaluate for anxiety, depression, other mental health
• Psychosocial	E.g., young children, complex family dynamics
• Thoughts & beliefs	Biomedical bias? Coping style? Religiosity?
3. Negotiate decision	If impasse, accept and move on to other areas where collaboration can be achieved

to be reached on the way forward. The article concludes by counseling clinicians what to do if the family continues to demand aggressive life-sustaining treatment despite following the framework. Clinicians are advised to avoid harassing the patient/family about the advance care plan, and to move on to an area that can be agreed on, such as symptom control.

CONCLUSIONS

In general, shared decision making is important in modern health care as most decisions are preference sensitive. This is especially true in cancer medicine, when there are multiple competing options with uncertain unpredictable outcomes. Careful elicitation of the patient's understanding, mood, and psychosocial factors is needed to understand the choice and to guide it. However, the clinician needs to be aware of the many cognitive biases that operate when humans make complex decisions in the face of uncertainty and how to limit their impact. The high stakes, high emotion setting of advanced cancer can be a challenge for SDM when patients/families make requests for treatment that may not be in the best interests of the patient's or conducive to promote quality of life.

This is the ultimate dilemma for PCM. It is fitting to end with Prof. Norelle Lickiss' cogent words, "yet we may fail to grasp the complexity of personhood, because of inadequate reflection and a deficient philosophy. An ecological view of the person remedies this by giving him or her a framework: a person has a complex personal environment, a unique inheritance (cultural and biological) and a unique personal history. He or she is not a closed ecological system for he or she can reach out in hope - towards what is other" [16].

ACKNOWLEDGMENTS AND DISCLOSURES

No conflicts of interest reported.

REFERENCES

1. Ostermann J, Brown DS, van Til JA, Bansback N, Legare F, Marshall DA, Bewtra M. 2019. Support Tools for Preference-Sensitive Decisions in Healthcare: Where Are We? Where Do We Go? How Do We Get There? Patient 12(5): 439–443.
2. Quill TE, Holloway RG. 2012. Evidence, Preferences, Recommendations: Finding the Right Balance in Patient Care. New England Journal of Medicine 366 (18): 1653–1655.
3. Elwyn G, Frosch D, Thomson R, Joseph-Williams N, Lloyd A, Kinnersley P, Cording E, Tomson D, Dodd C, Rollnick S, Edwards A, Barry M. 2012.

Shared Decision Making: A Model for Clinical Practice. Journal of General Internal Medicine 27 (10): 1361–1367.

4. Kluger J, Park A. 2013. The Angelina Effect. Time Magazine. May 27, 2013.

5. Bruera E, Sweeney C, Calder K, Palmer L, Benisch-Tolley S. 2001. Patient Preferences versus Physician Perceptions of Treatment Decisions in Cancer Care. Journal of Clinical Oncology 19 (11): 2883–2885.

6. Verma AA, Razak F, Detsky AS. 2014. Understanding Choice: Why Physicians Should Learn Prospect Theory. Journal of the American Medical Association 311 (6): 571–572.

7. Christakis NA, Iwashyna TJ. 1998. Attitude and Self-reported Practice Regarding Prognostication in a National Sample of Internists. Archives of Internal Medicine 158 (21): 2389–2395.

8. Shih YT, Chien CR. 2017. A Review of Cost Communication in Oncology: Patient Attitude, Provider Acceptance, and Outcome Assessment. Cancer 123 (6): 928–939.

9. McNeil BJ, Pauker SG, Sox HC Jr., Tversky A. 1982. On the Elicitation of Preferences for Alternative Therapies. New England Journal of Medicine 306 (21): 1259–1262.

10. Glare P, Fridman I, Ashton-James CE. 2018. Choose Your Words Wisely: The Impact of Message Framing on Patients' Responses to Treatment Advice. International Review of Neurobiology 139: 159–190.

11. Higgins ET. 1997. Beyond Pleasure and Pain. American Psychologist 52 (12): 1280–1300.

12. Avnet T, Higgins ET. 2006. How Regulatory Fit Affects Value in Consumer Choices and Opinions. Journal of Marketing Research 18 (February): 1–10.

13. Fridman I, Epstein AS, Higgins ET. 2015. Appropriate Use of Psychology in Patient-Physician Communication: Influencing Wisely. JAMA Oncology 1 (6): 725–726.

14. Fridman I, Glare PA, Stabler SM, Epstein AS, Wiesenthal A, Leblanc TW, Tory Higgins E. 2018. Information Framing Reduces Initial Negative Attitudes in Cancer Patients' Decisions about Hospice Care. Journal of Pain and Symptom Management 55 (6): 1540–1545.

15. Quill TE, Arnold R, Back AL. 2009. Discussing Treatment Preferences with Patients Who *Want* "Everything." Annals of Internal Medicine 151 (5): 345–349.

16. Lickiss JN. 2001. Approaching Cancer Pain Relief. European Journal of Pain 5 (Suppl A): 5–14.

SHARED DECISION MAKING FOR OTHER GENERAL CONDITIONS

W. James Appleyard, MA, MD, FRCP[a] and Jon Snaedal, MD[b]

ABSTRACT

Shared decision making based on clinical evidence and the patient's informed preferences improves patient knowledge and ability to participate in their care with improvement to those with long-term health problems.

A common ground between the patient and the physician is achieved through empathic communication skills with the provision of evidence-based information about options, outcomes, and uncertainties, together with decision support counseling and a systematic approach to recording and implementing patient's preferences.

It is important to recognize that the complexities of the clinical decision-making process with the confounding variables create difficulties in obtaining and measuring reproducible outcomes.

Keywords: shared decision making, chronic diseases, noncommunicable disease, therapeutic alliance, person-centered care, children

Correspondence Address: Prof. W. James Appleyard, Thimble Hall Blean Common, Kent CT2 9JJ, United Kingdom

E-mail: jimappleyard2510@aol.com

THE OVERLAPPING SPECTRUM OF COMMUNICABLE AND NONCOMMUNICABLE CHRONIC DISEASES

The World Health Organization (WHO) has called for a fundamental paradigm shift in the way health services are funded, managed, and delivered to urgently

---

[a] *Board Advisor and Former President, International College of Person Centered Medicine; Former President, World Medical Association; President, International Association of Medical Colleges*
[b] *President, International College of Person Centered Medicine; Professor of Geriatric Medicine, Landspitali University Hospital, Reykjavik, Iceland*

meet the challenges being faced by health systems around the world [1]. One key driver of this paradigm shift is the change in the nature of health care problems. Once focused on the management of infectious diseases, the burden of health care in the 21st century is shifting toward noncommunicable diseases, mental health, and injuries. Many of these conditions are chronic, requiring long-term care, with patients commonly suffering from multimorbidities, all of which adds to escalating health care costs.

Developing more integrated people-centered care systems is seen as the way forward in this situation, and empowering and engaging people is a key strategy in achieving this. Harnessing individuals and families is important to achieve better clinical outcomes in noncommunicable and chronic diseases through coproduction of care. To enable coproduction of care, patients and families need health education, participation in shared clinical decision making, and learning how to practice self-management. This paper focuses on the second aim: shared decision making (SDM).

Before discussing SDM further, it is worth noting that many noncommunicable chronic diseases, including cardiovascular disease and chronic respiratory disease, are linked to communicable diseases in either etiology or susceptibility to severe outcomes [1]. Similarly, many cancers, including some with global impact such as cancer of the cervix, liver, oral cavity, and stomach, have been shown to have an infectious etiology. In developing countries, infections are known to be the cause of about one-fifth of cancer. Strong population-based services to control infectious diseases through prevention, including immunization (e.g., vaccines against hepatitis B, human papillomavirus, measles, rubella, influenza, pertussis, and poliomyelitis), diagnosis and treatment. and control strategies will reduce both the burden and the impact of noncommunicable diseases.

There is also a high risk of infectious disease acquisition and susceptibility in people with preexisting noncommunicable diseases. High rates of other cancers in developing countries that are linked to infections or infestations include herpes virus and HIV in Kaposi sarcoma, and liver flukes in cholangiocarcinoma. Some significant disabilities such as blindness, deafness, cardiac defects, and intellectual impairment can derive from preventable infectious causes.

THE EVIDENCE BASE FOR SDM IN NONCOMMUNICABLE DISEASE

In a literature search, the principles of shared decision making (SDM) were well documented [2–4]. However, there is no consensus about its application and effectiveness in the different areas of clinical practice.

In 1982, the Presidential Commission in the United States published its seminal report, *Making Health Care Decisions* [5], advocating for informed medical decision making shared between the patient and health care providers that is sensitive to patient values and goals. The idea draws on and reemphasizes the principles of person-centered care leading to a greater focus on the skills required and the ability to use these skills in everyday clinical practice.

HOW TO PRACTICE SDM

Shared decision making is based on the available clinical evidence and the patient's informed preferences. This dialogue improves patient knowledge and ability to participate in their care with the consequent improvement to those with long-term health problems. This more "personalized" planning of a patient's care is a collaborative process involving a conversation, or series of conversations, in which jointly agreed goals and actions are formulated for managing the patient's problems [6].

It involves the provision of evidence-based information about options, outcomes, and uncertainties, together with decision support counseling and a systematic approach to recording and implementing patient's preferences.

Clinicians and patients work together to select tests, treatments, management, or support packages, based on clinical evidence and the patient's informed preferences [7].

There are many different approaches for achieving "common ground," which all have a similar emphasis on the importance of creating a formulation or integrated synthesis of the clinical and personal data about the patient that support the diagnosis and serve as a bridge between assessment and the creation of a treatment plan.

Each approach also focuses on the value of a written narrative that captures the essence of the understanding and the importance of dialogue between the patient and the physician that is the foundation of common ground [8].

Disagreements must be acknowledged and reconciled in the process; without this, the therapeutic alliance central to healing relationships is absent and a meaningful treatment plan based on shared decision making cannot be achieved. Synthesizing the data collected in assessment into insight and understanding that can help to establish shared understanding and common ground is essential.

Translating that understanding into effective, individualized and culturally sensitive/informed treatment plans is at the heart of person-centered care.

SDM IN CHRONIC DISEASES

A Cochrane review of "personalized" care planning for adults with chronic and long-term conditions identified 19 studies, mainly in primary care, involving a total of 10,856 participants, intended to support behavior change among patients, involving either face-to-face or telephone support [9]. Diseases included diabetes, mental health, heart failure, end-stage renal disease, asthma, and one study on various chronic conditions. In detail, nine studies involved using measurements of glycosylated hemoglobin (HbA1c) in patients with diabetes and revealed a small positive effect in favor of personalized care planning compared to usual care; six studies relating to hypertension measured improvement in systolic blood pressure, favoring personalized care though there was no significant effect on diastolic blood pressure; one study involved people with asthma reported that personalized care planning led to improvements in lung function and asthma control; six studies measured depression and a small effect in favor of personalized care (moderate quality evidence) was found.

There were no consistent findings in ten studies, which used various patient-reported measures of health status (or health-related quality of life), including both generic health status measures and condition-specific ones.

Nine studies looked at the effect of personalized care on self-management capabilities using a variety of outcome measures, but they focused primarily on self-efficacy. The pooled results from five studies that measured self-efficacy gave a small positive result in favor of personalized care planning.

No evidence was found of adverse effects due to personalized care planning.

The effects of personalized care planning were greater when more stages of the care planning cycle were completed, when contacts between patients and health professionals were more frequent, and when the patient's usual clinician was involved in the process.

The authors concluded that personalized care planning leads to improvements in certain indicators of physical and psychological health status, and people's capability to self-manage their condition when compared to usual care. The effects are not large, but they appear greater when the intervention is more comprehensive, more intensive, and better integrated into routine care [10].

SDM IN CHILDHOOD

SDM in pediatrics is necessarily different than SDM in adult medicine. Specifically, in pediatrics, the extent to which the child as a patient is involved in decision making varies significantly [11]. Some child patients such as the young, the immature, those with severe cognitive difficulties, sedated patients in the ICU, etc. may be wholly left out of decision making, whereas other patients including older adolescents, those with chronic illness, the more mature may be the primary decision makers in their own care. With such a wide array of roles for pediatric patients in their own care, any conceptualization of SDM in pediatrics must be flexible enough to allow for such varied inclusion of the children in the decision-making team. Fifteen research studies where this heterogeneity was high were included in a meta-analysis, which revealed SDM interventions significantly improved knowledge and reduced decisional conflict with a nonsignificant trend toward increased parental satisfaction.

In pediatric practice the gold standard is the best interest of the child patient, but debate continues regarding the weight that may be given to the interests of parents and other siblings. Because minors lack legal authority to provide informed consent for treatment except in specific circumstances as defined by national law, SDM in pediatrics must necessarily include the parent or legal guardian.

Because parents will identify as the children's protectors, they are often reluctant to consider less aggressive goals of care than are surrogates of adult patients. Furthermore, because there is often a sense that children "have not yet really lived" parents may be more focused on any chance of survival regardless of the cost in terms of time, pain and suffering, cost, etc. than are surrogates as outcomes for such research. Researchers have considered an array of outcomes, including parental satisfaction, health care team satisfaction, decisional regret, lack of legal action, hospital length of stay, overall admission cost, adherence to predetermined communication guidelines, etc. However, there remains disagreement regarding the specific goals in SDM and how best to assess whether the goals were met in any given case. The authors conclude that there is not currently sufficient data to support an evidence-based holistic conceptualization of SDM in pediatrics.

CONCLUSIONS

The application of conceptual models through the creation of narrative formulations can significantly contribute to ensuring that care is person centered. Synthesizing the data collected in assessment into insight and understanding that can help to establish shared understanding and common ground is essential. Translating that understanding into effective, individualized, and culturally sensitive/informed treatment plans is at the heart of person-centered care.

ACKNOWLEDGMENTS AND DISCLOSURES

No conflicts of interest declared.

REFERENCES

1. WHO. 2015. Global Strategy on People Centered Integrated Health Services, World Health Organization, Geneva.

2. Coulter A. 1997. Partnerships with Patients: The Pros and Cons of Shared Clinical Decision-Making. Journal of Health Services Research & Policy 2: 112–121.
3. Coulter A, Harter M, Moumjid-Ferdjaoui N, Perestelo-Perez L, van der Weijden T 2015. European Experience with Shared Decision Making. International Journal of Person Centered Medicine 5: 9–14.
4. Elwyn G, Frosch D, Thomson R, Joseph-Williams N, Lloyd A, Kinnersley P. 2012. Shared Decision Making: A Model for Clinical Practice. Journal of General Internal Medicine 27: 1361–1367.
5. President's Commission for the Study of Ethical Problems in Medicine, Biomedical, Behavioral Research (US). 1982. Making health care decisions. President's Commission for the Study of Ethical Problems in Medicine and Biomedical and Behavioral Research.
6. Elwyn GJ, Edwards A, Kinnersley P. 1999. Shared Decision Making in Primary Care: The Neglected Second Half of the Consultation. British Journal of General Practice 49: 477–482.
7. Adams N. 2012. Finding Common Ground: The Role of Integrative Diagnosis and Treatment Planning as a Pathway to Person-Centered Care. International Journal of Person Centered Medicine 2: 173–178.
8. Bieber C, Nicolai J, Hartmann M, Blumenstiel K, Ringel N, Schneider A, Haerter M, Eich W, Log A. 2009. Training Physicians in Shared Decision Making – Who Can Be Reached and What Is Achieved? Patient Education and Counselling7: 48–54.
9. Coulter A, Entwistle VA, Eccles A, Ryan S, Shepperd S, Perera R. 2015. Personalised Care Planning for Adults with Chronic or Long-Term Health Conditions. Cochrane Database of Systematic Reviews Issue 3.
10. Kennedy A, Bower P, Reeves D, Blakeman T, Bowen R, Chew-Graham C, on behalf of the Salford National Institute for Health Research Gastrointestinal Programme Grant Research Group. 2013. Implementation of Self-management Support for Long-Term Conditions in Routine Primary Care Settings: Cluster Randomised Controlled Trial. British Medical Journal 346: 2882.
11. Kon AA, Morrison W. 2018. Shared Decision-Making in Pediatric Practice: A Broad View. Pediatrics 142 (Suppl 3): S129–S132.

INTERPROFESSIONAL COLLABORATION FOR PERSON-CENTERED CARE

Tesfamicael Ghebrehiwet, PhD, MPHa

ABSTRACT

Interprofessional collaboration (IPC) occurs when health workers with varying educational preparation and skills work together to deliver quality health services – as no single health professional can have all the required knowledge and skills. Governments and health policy makers are always looking for better ways of delivering care and IPC offers a smart solution to do this. Interprofessional education (IPE), an related concept, is a prerequisite in preparing a "collaborative practice-ready" health workforce that is better prepared to respond to local health needs. In interprofessional education, health workers, at some point during their training, learn together in order to work together.

Keywords: interprofessional collaboration, collaborative practice, interprofessional education, interdisciplinary health team, health care team approach

Correspondence Address: Dr. Tesfa Ghebrehiwet, 27 Kinkora Manor, NW, Calgary, AB. T3R 1N7, Canada

E-mail: tesfa@shaw.ca

INTRODUCTION

The World Health Organization defines interprofessional collaboration (IPC) as "multiple health workers from different professional backgrounds working together with patients, families, caregivers and communities to deliver the highest quality of care" [1]. In the current landscape of global shortage of human and financial resources and fragmented health systems, interprofessional collaboration offers a promising solution to strengthening health systems to meet complex health needs, and improving health outcomes [2, 3].

---

a Board Director, International College of Person Centered Medicine; Former Policy Officer, International Council of Nurses, Geneva, Switzerland

In an era of increased consumer demand, shifting disease patterns and increasing chronic diseases, providing quality, cost-effective care, requires a coordinated approach by the various health professionals. IPC can be effectively introduced in the delivery of comprehensive primary health care services as well as for providing episodic and continuous care of chronic conditions.

Interprofessional education, an interrelated concept, is prerequisite in preparing a "collaborative practice-ready" health workforce that is better prepared to respond to local health needs [1]. In interprofessional education, health workers, at some point during their training, learn together in order to work together.

INTERPROFESSIONAL COLLABORATION AND COMMUNICATION

Interprofesssional collaboration is essential for improving access to patient-centered care. Interprofessional communication is a key element of collaborative practice. Effective communication facilitates information sharing and decision making. Interdisciplinary approach combines a joint effort with a common goal from all disciplines involved. In collaborative practice health professionals [4–6]:

- cooperate and assume complementary roles,
- share responsibility for problem solving and decision making to formulate and implement patient care plans, and
- increase awareness of team members' knowledge and skills, leading to continued improvement in decision making.

The pooling of specialized services leads to integrated interventions and avoids fragmentation of care. The plan of care takes into account the multiple professional inputs into assessments and treatment regimens. Interprofessional communication relies on transparent, honest interactions between the different health professionals.

A CONTINUUM OF CARE

The division of labor among medical, nursing, and other health professionals highlights the importance of interdependent care because no single professional can have the expertise and knowledge to provide a continuum of care [7]. At the center of interprofessional collaboration is the person who has health problems and who should be an active partner in care. And this is the essence of person-centered care.

Interprofessional collaboration is applicable to all stages of the health care delivery continuum, including health promotion, disease prevention, detection, treatment, and rehabilitation. The key principles of IPC include [8]:

- Focus should be on the patient;
- Health needs of the population should drive the services offered;
- Health outcomes should be tracked for effectiveness and quality;
- Access should be provided where and when it is needed;
- Shared decision making by professions with different skills and knowledge will foster creativity and innovation; and
- Effective communication facilitates information-sharing and decision making.

INTERPROFESSIONAL EDUCATION (IPE)

The World Health Organization [1] identifies IPE as the process by which a group of more than two profession-specific students from health-related occupations with different educational backgrounds learn together during certain periods of their education with interaction as an important goal. Interdisciplinary team approach is the hallmark of positive outcomes for the health of patients, families, and communities. However, a number of reports affirm interprofessional collaboration does not come naturally to health professionals and require a paradigm shift in educational programs [9, 10]. As Frenk et al. [11] have affirmed, the excessive focus on hospital-based education that is segregated into professional silos does not prepare health professionals for team work, and for leadership skills in the 21st-century health services.

In general, most health care organizations and health profession educational institutions devote little or no time and resources to promote interdisciplinary collaboration and functioning. In fact, the different health profession training programs take place in different buildings, and in different colleges or schools often within the same campus. Often similar courses are taught separately for the different health professions, adding to the silo approach of educational institutions [12].

Efforts to improve patient safety and quality are often jeopardized by barriers in communication and collaboration. Interprofessional education (IPE) is key for IPC and provides a promising solution to work in smart and efficient ways. Thus, to implement IPC health profession curriculum needs to be transformed to include IPE with collaboration and communication as core competencies.

ELEMENTS OF INTERPROFESSIONAL COLLABORATION

Health care professionals are not always ready to embrace true team practice. In order to understand collaborative practice, we first need to appreciate the basic elements of the team approach in health care. Regardless of the team model, all have three basic elements in common [13]:

- Multiple providers: no single profession can meet all patients' needs.
- Service coordination/collaboration: to ensure continuity and avoid fragmentation of care.
- Communication: in order to provide comprehensive, efficient, and patient-centered care.

Beyond multiple providers sharing information to coordinate comprehensive care, health professionals engaged in collaborative practice need to work together in defining and achieving common goals, develop strong team identity and mutual respect, and view their actions as interdependent.

BARRIERS TO INTERPROFESSIONAL COLLABORATION AND COMMUNICATION

Communication and collaboration do not always occur in clinical settings. Social, relational, and organizational structures contribute to communication failures that can contribute to adverse clinical events and outcomes [14, 15].

Some barriers to interprofessional collaboration that need to be overcome include [14, 16]:

- Additional time; perceived loss of autonomy;
- Lack of confidence or trust in decisions of others;
- Clashing perceptions; territorialism; hierarchy; and
- Lack of awareness of the education, knowledge, and skills of other disciplines.

Most of these barriers can be overcome with an open attitude, mutual respect, and trust. IPE offers an upstream solution to addressing the barriers.

CONSEQUENCES OF POOR COLLABORATION AND COMMUNICATION

Medical errors that threaten patient safety can occur in virtually all stages of diagnosis and treatment. Improvements in patient safety can be achieved when the workforce fully participates in organizational processes, safety systems, improvement initiatives, and is trained in the roles and services for which they are accountable. Poor interprofessional collaboration and communication can put patient safety at risk related to [17, 18]:

- lack of critical information,
- misinterpretation of information,
- unclear orders over the telephone, and
- overlooked changes in patient status.

In fact collaboration and communication failures are the leading root causes for medication errors, delayed treatment, misdiagnosis, and patient injury or death.

BENEFITS OF COLLABORATION AND COMMUNICATION

The benefits to patients, staff, and the health care delivery system provide a compelling reason to implement interprofessional collaboration at all levels of health care delivery. Effective IPCC can lead to positive patient outcomes, improved staff morale, and patient satisfaction related to the following issues [14, 19]:

- improved information flow,
- better patient outcomes,
- improved patient safety,
- enhanced employee morale,
- increased patient and family satisfaction, and
- decreased length of hospital stay.

Effective communication encourages collaboration, fosters teamwork, and helps prevent medical errors.

CONCLUSIONS

Interprofessional collaboration is key to quality care and patient safety as no single health care provider can have all the knowledge and skills to meet all the patient's needs. Interprofessional communication enhances collaboration and helps prevent medical errors. Health care organizations need to offer a safe practice environment with programs that foster IPCC and improve patient outcomes. Interprofessional education is an integral element of collaboration and ensuring that health professionals are "collaborative practice ready." This is achieved by learning together in order to work together.

ACKNOWLEDGMENTS AND DISCLOSURES

No conflicts of interest are declared.

REFERENCES

1. World Health Organization. 2010. Framework for Action on Interprofessional Education & Collaborative Practice. Geneva: WHO. Available at: http:// whqlibdoc.who.int/hq/2010/WHO_HRH_HPN_10.3_eng.pdf?ua=1
2. Mickan S, Hoffman SJ, Nasmith L. 2010. Collaborative Practice in a Global Health Context: Common Themes from Developed and Developing Countries. World Health Organization Study Group on Interprofessional Education and Collaborative Practice. Journal of Interprofessional Care 24 (5): 492–502.
3. Zwarenstein M, Goldman J, Reeves S. 2009. Interprofessional Collaboration: Effects of Practice-Based Interventions on Professional Practice and Healthcare Outcomes. Cochrane Database of Systematic Reviews Issue 3. Art. No.: CD000072. Doi: 10.1002/14651858.CD000072.pub2
4. Fagin CM. 1992. Collaboration between Nurses and Physicians: No Longer a Choice. Academic Medicine 67 (5): 295–303.
5. Baggs J, Schmitt MH. 1988. Collaboration between Nurses and Physicians. Image: the Journal of Nursing Scholarship 20 (3): 145–149.
6. Christensen C, Larson JR. 1993. Collaborative Medical Decision Making. Medical Decision Making 13 (4): 339–346.
7. Sicotte C, Pinealut R, Lambert J. 1993. Medical Interdependence as a Determinant of Use of Clinical Resources. Health Services Research 28 (5): 599–609.
8. EICP Steering Committee. 2005. The Principles and Framework for Interdisciplinary Collaboration in Primary Health Care, EICP Initiative, Ottawa.
9. Bhutta Z , Chen L, Cohen J, Crisp N, Evans T, Fineberg H, Frenk J, Garcia P, Horton R, Ke Y, Kelley P, Kistnasamy B, Meleis A, David Naylor D, Pablos-Mendez A, Reddy S, Scrimshaw S, Sepulveda J, Serwadda D, Zurayk, H. (2010). Education of Health Professionals for the 21st Century: A Global Independent Commission. Lancet 375 (9721): 1137–1138.
10. Institute of Medicine. 2003. Health Professions Education: A Bridge to Quality, National Academy Press, Washington, DC.
11. Frenk J, Chen L, Bhutta Z, Cohen J, Crisp N, Timothy Evans T, Fineberg H, Garcia P, Ke Y, Kelley P, Kistnasamy B, Meleis A, Naylor D, Pablos-Mendez A, Reddy S, Scrimshaw S, Sepulveda J, David Serwadda D, Zurayk, H. (2010). Health Professionals for a New Century: Transforming Education to Strengthen Health Systems in an Interdependent World. The Lancet Commissions 376 (9756): 1923–1958.
12. Drinka TJK, Clark PG. 2000. Health Care Teamwork: Interdisciplinary Practice and Teaching, Auburn House, Connecticut.

13. International Council of Nurses. 2004. Collaborative Practice in the 21st Century. Developed by Madrean Schober and Nancy MacKay, for the International Council of Nurses. Geneva.
14. Liaw SY, Zhou WT, Lau TC, Siau C, Chan SW. 2014. An Interprofessional Communication Training Using Simulation to Enhance Safe Care for a Deteriorating Patient. Nurse Education Today 34 (2): 259–264.
15. Rice K, Zwarenstein M, Conn LG, Kenaszchuk C, Russell A, Reeves S. 2010. An Intervention to Improve Interprofessional Collaboration and Communications: A Comparative Qualitative Study. Journal of Interprofessional Care 24 (4): 350e361.
16. Nadzam DM. 2009. Nurses' Role in Communication and Patient Safety. Journal of Nursing Care Quality 24 (3): 184e188.
17. Kate F. 2018. The Joint Commission's Hospital National Patient Safety Goals for 2018. Healthcare, Jan.4, 2018. Available at: https://www.compass-clinical.com/the-joint-commission-national-patient-safety-goals-for-2018
18. Australian Commission on Safety and Quality in Health Care. 2011. National Safety and Quality Health Services. Available at: https://www.safetyandquality.gov.au/wp-content/uploads/2011/01/NSQHS-Standards-Sept2011.pdf
19. Shortell SM, Zimmerman JE, Rousseau DM, Gillies RR, Wagner DP, Draper EA, Knaus WA, Duffy J. 1994. The Performance of Intensive Care Units: Does Good Management Make a Difference? Medical Care 32 (5): 508–525.

www.ingramcontent.com/pod-product-compliance
Lightning Source LLC
Chambersburg PA
CBHW060315220326
41598CB00027B/4329